Growing Older

Quality of life in old age

Growing Older

Series Editor: Alan Walker

The objective of this series is to showcase the major outputs from the ESRC Growing Older programme and to provide research insights which will result in improved practice and enhanced and extended quality of life for older people.

It is well-known that people are living longer but until now very little attention has been given to the factors that determine the quality of life experienced by older people. This important new series will be vital reading for a broad audience of policymakers, social gerontologists, nurses, social workers, sociologists and social geographers as well as advanced undergraduate and postgraduate students in these disciplines.

Series titles include:

Ann Bowling *Ageing Well*

Joanne Cook, Tony Maltby and Lorna Warren *Older Women's Lives*

Maria Evandrou and Karen Glaser *Family, Work and Quality of Life for Older People*

Mary Maynard, Haleh Afshar, Myfanwy Franks and Sharon Wray *Women in Later Life*

Sheila Peace, Caroline Holland and Leonie Kellaher *Environment and Identity in Later Life*

Thomas Scharf, Chris Phillipson and Allison E Smith *Ageing in the City*

Christina Victor, Sasha Scambler and John Bond *The Social World of Older People*

Alan Walker (ed) *Growing Older in Europe*

Alan Walker and Catherine Hagan Hennessy (eds) *Growing Older*: quality of life in old age

Alan Walker and Catherine Hagan Hennessy (eds) *Understanding Quality of Life in Old Age*

Growing Older

Quality of life in old age

edited by
Alan Walker and
Catherine Hagan Hennessy

Open University Press

Open University Press
McGraw-Hill Education
McGraw-Hill House
Shoppenhangers Road
Maidenhead
Berkshire
England
SL6 2QL
email: enquiries@openup.co.uk
world wide web: www.openup.co.uk

and Two Penn Plaza, New York, NY 10121-2289, USA

First published 2004

A catalogue record of this book is available from the British Library

ISBN 0335 21507 6 (pb) 0335 21508 4 (hb)

Library of Congress Cataloging-in-Publication Data
CIP data applied for

Typeset by YHT Ltd, London
Printed in the UK by MPG Books Ltd, Bodmin, Cornwall

Contents

Contributors   vi

Preface   ix

1 Introducing the Growing Older Programme on extending quality of life
Alan Walker   1

2 Quality of life in old age from the perspectives of older people
Zahava Gabriel and Ann Bowling   14

3 Ethnic inequalities
James Nazroo, Madhavi Bajekal, David Blane and Ini Grewal 35

4 Environment, identity and old age: Quality of life or a life of quality?
Leonie Kellaher, Sheila M. Peace and Caroline Holland   60

5 Poverty and social exclusion: Growing older in deprived urban neighbourhoods
Thomas Scharf, Chris Phillipson and Allison E. Smith   81

6 Loneliness in later life
Christina R. Victor, Sasha J. Scambler, John Bond and Ann Bowling   107

7 Older men: Their health behaviours and partnership status
Kate Davidson and Sara Arber   127

8 A participatory approach to older women's quality of life
Joanne Cook, Tony Maltby and Lorna Warren   149

9 Social support and ethnicity in old age
Jabeer Butt and Jo Moriarty   167

10 The meaning of grandparenthood and its contribution to the quality of life of older people
Lynda Clarke and Ceridwen Roberts   188

11 Frailty and institutional life
Susan Tester, Gill Hubbard, Murna Downs, Charlotte MacDonald and Joan Murphy   209

12 Conclusion
Catherine Hagan Hennessy   225

Bibliography   230

Index   260

Contributors

Sara Arber, Professor and Head of School of Human Sciences, Department of Sociology, University of Surrey
www.soc.surrey.ac.uk/sara_arber.htm

Madhavi Bajekal, Research Director, National Centre for Social Research
www.natcen.ac.uk/natcen

David Blane, Reader in Medical Sociology, Imperial College London
www.ic.ac.uk

John Bond, Professor of Social Gerontology and Health Services Research, Centre for Health Services Research, University of Newcastle
www.ncl.ac.uk/chsr/staff

Ann Bowling, Professor of Health Services Research, Department of Primary Care and Population Sciences, University College London
www.ucl.ac.uk/primcare-popsci/aps/

Jabeer Butt, Deputy Director, REU
www.reu.org.uk

Lynda Clarke, Course Director/Senior Lecturer, London School of Hygiene and Tropical Medicine
www.lshtm.ac.uk/cps/staff/lclarke.html

Joanne Cook, Research Fellow, European Forum on Population Ageing Research, Department of Sociological Studies, University of Sheffield
www.shef.ac.uk/socst/staff/j_cook.htm

Kate Davidson, Lecturer in Social Policy and Sociology, Department of Sociology and Co-Director of the Centre for Research on Ageing and Gender (CRAG), University of Surrey
www.soc.surrey.ac.uk/kate_davidson.htm

Murna Downs, Professor in Dementia Studies, Bradford Dementia Group, University of Bradford
www.brad.ac.uk/acad/health/bdg.htm

Zahava Gabriel, Health Outcomes Analyst, Heron Evidence Development
www.herongroup.co.uk/

Ini Grewal, Senior Researcher, National Centre for Social Research
www.natcen.ac.uk/

Catherine Hagan Hennessy, Deputy Director ESRC Growing Older Programme, Department of Sociological Studies, University of Sheffield
www.shef.ac.uk/socst/staff/c_hennessy.htm

Caroline Holland, Research Associate, School of Health and Social Welfare, The Open University
www.open.ac.uk/shsw/

Gill Hubbard, Senior Research Fellow, General Practice & Primary Care, University of Glasgow
www.gla.ac.uk/departments/generalpractice

Leonie Kellaher, Director of Centre for Environmental and Social Studies in Ageing (CESSA), London Metropolitan University
www.londonmet.ac.uk/pg-prospectus-2003/research/centres/cessa.cfm

Charlotte MacDonald, Independent Research Consultant and Honorary Fellow, University of Stirling

Tony Maltby, Senior Lecturer in Social Policy, Institute for Applied Social Studies, University of Birmingham
www.spsw.bham.ac.uk/

Jo Moriarty, Research Fellow, Social Care Workforce Research Unit, King's College London
www.kcl.ac.uk

Joan Murphy, Research Speech and Language Therapist, Department of Psychology, University of Stirling
www.aacscotland.com

James Nazroo, Professor of Medical Sociology, University College London
www.ucl.ac.uk/medical-sociology

Sheila M. Peace, Sub-Dean and Director of Research, School of Health and Social Welfare, The Open University
www.open.ac.uk/shsw

Chris Phillipson, Professor of Applied Social Studies and Social Gerontology and Director of the Institute of Ageing, Keele University
www.keele.ac.uk/depts/so/csg/index.htm

Ceridwen Roberts, Senior Research Fellow, Department of Social Policy and Social Work, University of Oxford
www.apsoc.ox.ac.uk/

Sasha J. Scambler, Lecturer in Sociology, University of Surrey Roehampton
www.roehampton.ac.uk

Thomas Scharf, Reader in Social Gerontology and Director of the Centre for Social Gerontology, Keele University
www.keele.ac.uk/depts/so/csg/index.htm

Allison E. Smith, Research Assistant and doctoral student, Centre for Social Gerontology, Keele University

Susan Tester, Senior Lecturer in Social Policy, Department of Applied Social Science, University of Stirling
www.stir.ac.uk/Departments/HumanSciences/AppSocSci/SSP/staff/Stester.htm

Alan Walker, Professor of Social Policy, Department of Sociological Studies, University of Sheffield, and Director of the ESRC Growing Older Programme
www.shef.ac.uk/socst/staff/a_walker.htm
www.shef.ac.uk/uni/projects/gop/

Lorna Warren, Lecturer, Department of Sociological Studies, University of Sheffield
www.shef.ac.uk/socst/staff/l_warren.htm

Christina R. Victor, Professor and Dean for Postgraduate Teaching and Learning, Department of Public Health Sciences, St George's Hospital Medical School
www.sghms.ac.uk/Departments/phs.htm

Preface

The Growing Older (GO) Programme spanned seven years from conception to formal completion and we want to gratefully acknowledge the many contributions that have been made to it along the way. First and foremost is the Economic and Social Research Council (ESRC) which not only funded the programme in its entirety but was also responsible for taking the initiative in the first place. The Research Priorities Board of the ESRC was the one that approved the initial proposal and eventually the programme itself and which oversaw its implementation. The programme has had excellent support from the ESRC, from the Anthropology, Linguistics, Psychology, Health and Sociology Research Area led by Ros Rouse; from Kathy Ham and Iain Stewart of the External Relations Division; and from a series of ESRC programme officers including Faye Auty and Naomi Beaumont at the beginning and Shabnam Khan at the end.

Then there are the project researchers, among whom are some of the UK's leading social scientists in this field but, also, many new faces who will form the next generation of outstanding social scientists. There are 96 researchers associated with the programme and their cooperation has been an essential feature of its success. They have responded happily (for the most part) to the seemingly endless series of requests from the programme office. It has been a privilege to work with this high calibre group of social scientists. Of course they are responsible for the high quality of the research produced by the programme.

We also want to acknowledge the thousands of older people who took part in the GO projects as respondents and sometimes researchers or who contributed to the programme in other ways. We know that we owe them a duty to ensure that the best possible use is made of the results.

The programme Advisory Committee, chaired by Anthea Tinker, was a constant source of support and our thanks go to its members: Allan Bowman, Gillian Crosby, Leela Damodaran, Arthur Fleiss, Tessa Harding, Tom Hoyes, Paul Johnson, Carol Lupton, Robin Means, Terry Philpot, Martin Shreeve and Tony Warnes. Anthea Tinker could not have been a better chair in displaying a perfect balance of challenging questions and encouragement and in being a pleasure to work with. Arthur Fleiss was particularly helpful in creating links with policymakers and Tessa Harding with regard to non-governmental organisations working in the field of ageing. Shona Mullen and her colleagues at Open University Press have been extremely enthusiastic and supportive in getting this series underway.

Colleagues at the University of Sheffield have been very supportive towards the GO Programme, the Sheffield Institute for Studies on Ageing and the Department of Sociological Studies, especially Tim Booth who helped to ensure that it was properly staffed and located.

On a personal level we owe immense gratitude to our loved ones who bore the burden of the programme without any of its rewards. For Alan: Alison, Carol and Christopher Walker and for Catherine: Jamie Woolley, Elsie Broadbent and Otto von Mering, three ageless and inspiring friends.

Last but certainly not least, our sincere thanks to go the programme coordination team, including Alison Ball, Jo Levesley, Kristina Martimo and Roberta Nelson and, above all, to Marg Walker, for their major contributions to the whole GO Programme. This book is dedicated to Marg because not only did she prepare it for publication but, more importantly, she was the organisational lynchpin of the GO Programme itself.

Alan Walker
Catherine Hagan Hennessy
Department of Sociological Studies
University of Sheffield

To Marg Walker

1

Introducing the Growing Older Programme on extending quality life

Alan Walker

Introduction

There are three main purposes behind the production of this collection of chapters. It is intended, first of all, to present a state-of-the-art picture of quality of life in old age based on the most comprehensive programme of ageing research in the social sciences, or social gerontology, ever mounted in the UK. Selected from the Growing Older (GO) Programme, the chapters in this volume report some of the key findings to emerge from this major investigation. However, the ten contributions represent less than half of the projects that took part in the GO Programme. Therefore, obviously, they are a fraction of what might have been included if contemporary publishing conventions had allowed. The permutation of 10 from 24 was not an easy task because the quality of the projects is consistently very high. The findings from every project are published on the GO Programme website (www.shef.ac.uk/uni/projects/gop/) and in paper form and there is a summary booklet (Walker and Hennessy 2003) and a CD-ROM containing this material. The projects included here are not necessarily the best (or worst) but represent a cross-section covering the six main themes of the programme, which are also the main themes in quality of life among older people (see below). As such these chapters constitute the best available information in one volume on quality of life in old age and provide a comprehensive introduction to this vital topic for students, researchers, campaigners, practitioners, policy makers and, in fact, anyone interested in ageing and older people.

The second function of the book is to introduce the series that is based on the GO Programme. This is the first book in the series and is intended to serve as a taster of what is to follow. My (admittedly partial) view is that this will be a landmark series in social gerontology because of the high quality of the research it reports and the excellence of the researchers involved. There will be 11 other books in the series, including a novel thematic volume which engages all 24 projects.

Third, this book is intended to introduce the GO Programme itself. The ten core chapters report findings from it and the main part of this chapter is devoted to describing its background and orientation. Following this I will introduce the contents of the book itself.

Background, structure and operation of the GO programme

The origins of the GO Programme stretch back to 1995 and the Whitehall EQUAL initiative that posed the question how can the quality of people's lives be extended? The Economic and Social Research Council (ESRC) decided to develop a research programme on this topic, which I drafted. It was approved by the ESRC Council in May 1998 when £3.5 million was allocated. Following a two-stage commissioning process, 24 projects were selected for funding in May 1999. These projects are listed in Box 1.1 at the end of this chapter. The programme was established with two leading objectives:

1 To create a broad based multidisciplinary and co-ordinated programme of research on different aspects of quality of life in old age.

2 To try to contribute to the development of policies and practice in the field and, thereby, to the extension of quality life.

GO is an ESRC programme. Therefore its main aim is the generation of new high quality scientific knowledge, in this case on quality of life in old age. This means that the projects which make up the programme were selected on their scientific merit via the process of peer review. Thus, although the idea of the programme was developed by the ESRC, it was the responses of the social sciences community that determined its shape and content. As well as a scientific core, the GO Programme, unusually, has an explicit focus on policy and practice, so that it can try to have a tangible impact on extending the quality of older people's lives. The content of the programme was organised into six broad topic areas which cover all of the key aspects of quality of life in old age:

+ defining and measuring quality of life (5 projects)

+ inequalities in quality of life (5)

+ technology and the built environment (2)

+ healthy and active ageing (3)

+ family and support networks (5)

+ participation and activity in later life (4).

The first project commenced in October 1999 and the last in September 2000. The final project ended in April 2003 and the whole programme was completed in July 2004. When all of the projects were operational there were 96 researchers working on the programme, including many of the leading names in UK social gerontology. It has also proved to be a major training ground for new researchers in this field.

Programme overview

The GO Programme spanned seven years from conception to completion (although outputs will be generated for years to come and so 'completion' means the formal end of funding for the programme activities). What has been achieved by this huge research effort and financial investment? Recognising that the full impact of the scientific outputs from the programme will not be visible for some years, I want to highlight four major achievements.

First of all there is the essential scientific agenda of the GO Programme. The projects are of a remarkably consistent high quality and have generated many new insights into quality of life in old age: from measuring quality to understanding social exclusion, from the role of transport in the quality of later life to loneliness, and from environmental well-being to spirituality. Reports on the programme must refer to a large number of 'firsts' or 'most importants', for example: the creation of a new, theoretically-based, quality of life measuring tool; unique insights into stroke professionals and stroke survivors' perceptions of quality of life; the first representative study of what constitutes quality of life for older people; one of the few studies of older men's health; the most comprehensive research so far on black and ethnic minority ageing; the first representative study of the impact of exclusion an older people in deprived areas; the first research to identify transport as an independent component of quality of life; the first study to provide a comprehensive account of environmental well-being; a novel study of healthy ageing; the first UK investigations of the implication of multiple role occupancy for pensions; one of the very few studies anywhere on employment in later life to include those over pension ages; an innovative study of the impact of reminiscence on quality of life; the first research on spiritual belief among bereaved spouses; the first study to investigate why some frail older people resist help from the social services; unique research in grandparenting; the first national study of loneliness for nearly 50 years; the first research in the successful ageing priorities of older women from different ethnic groups; a unique study of participation among older women; an innovative project on learning and education in later life, and so on and so on. There is no doubting the variety and richness of this huge portfolio. As *The Guardian* journalist, Malcolm Dean put it:

> The inter-ministerial group on older people has had a national pro-gramme of its own for 'listening to older people', but with the completion of the ESRC programme, it can now turn from its parish library to the equivalent of the British Library, with a vast source of older people's views that should be able to answer many of the questions ministers want to ask.
>
> (Dean 2003: 2)

As well as the quality and quantity of the new knowledge that has been produced by the programme, it has also made a substantial contribution to research methods in this field, which is another important part of the legacy of GO. Examples include: the CASP 19 scale developed by David Blane and colleagues; the participative approaches used by Lorna Warren, Tony Maltby and their team; the *Talking Mats*™ used by Sue Tester and her team working with older people with dementia; the Wheel of Life developed by Sheila Peace and colleagues; the happy and sad faces used by Mary Gilhooly's team, and many more.

In sum, as far as the scientific achievements of the programme are concerned, GO has helped to put on the ageing research agenda or cement the existing place of some critically important topics and research methods. These include black and ethnic minority ageing, gender, spirituality, environmental well-being, political and community participation and participative research methods.

Second, among other things the original programme proposal emphasised the necessity of older people's perspectives and GO, more than previous British research, has been successful in researching and learning from older people's own attitudes, aspirations and preferences. This is a remarkable legacy for future researchers and a model for other countries. As the following chapters illustrate, the GO Programme has generated some amazingly rich and compelling data sets that are embedded in the lives of a wide variety of older people and the accounts based on them resonate with experiences and feelings.

Third, as noted already, unusually for a research council programme, a key objective of GO has been to try to influence policy and practice so that the research can contribute to the quality of older people's lives. Too often research appears to be conducted for its own sake but, in this field above many others, it is hard to justify the expenditure of public resources without tangible benefits for older people. Of course this begs huge questions about the connections between research and policy and practice. There cannot be a simple, straightforward relationship between research and policy and practice. Despite a widespread recognition of the desperate need for a more robust evidence base for policy and practice, there is still a great deal of confusion on both sides of this relationship. On the one hand, policymakers and practitioners often have unrealistic expectations of research (particularly regarding how quickly findings can be produced). On the other hand, researchers often hold false assumptions about the rationality of the policy process, that evidence leads to debate which leads to decisions, when nothing could be further from the truth.

In the absence of a rational model of decision making and when researchers cannot reasonably expect policymakers and practitioners to respond to their findings, the best way to influence decision makers is to permeate the context in which they work. This is the approach taken by the GO Programme. A policy/practice focus was introduced from the start and quite soon even the most reluctant and/or inexperienced researchers signed up to this mission. To try to inform policymakers we linked projects to civil servants working with the Inter-Ministerial Committee on Older People and held special seminars with key policymakers. The programme worked closely with the wider policy community, including NGOs. The media have been a particular target with help from the ESRC. The programme has produced accessible findings on each project and a specially commissioned booklet for policymakers (Dean 2003). While it cannot guarantee impact and influence, the programme has certainly tried to get its messages across.

Fourth, uniquely for a UK research programme, GO has had a very significant impact on European and international research agendas. For example, it led to the creation of the European Forum on Population Ageing Research under Framework Programme 5 (www.cordis.lu/fp5/home.html); it was part of a comparative study in five European countries (which will be reported in a subsequent volume); and it is a partner in the United Nation's Research Agenda on Ageing.

In sum there is no question that the programme's scientific outputs will play defining roles in many key areas of ageing research. But the question as to whether all this effort will improve older people's quality of life is still an open one.

Contents of the book

In this volume the authors of the main chapters draw from their research projects to report on the theme of quality of life in old age. Each chapter comprises a description of the research and its methods, an outline of the key findings and a discussion of their policy and, where relevant, practice implications. Together the following ten chapters constitute a unique state-of-the-art analysis of what determines quality in later life. Even in this selection from the full programme, the scope is huge – from the roles of neighbourhood and residence in quality of life to frailty in institutions; from ethnicity to loneliness; from gender to grandparenthood. Therefore there is a massive database contained in these pages and it deserves to be mined extensively by anyone and everyone interested in quality of life in old age. I will now highlight some of the main points from each chapter.

Chapter 2, by Zahava Gabriel and Ann Bowling, reports some of the qualitative results from their unique investigation into older people's own views about the quality of their lives. Their research was based on a large national survey of people aged 65 and over (999 participants) and follow-up interviews with 80 people chosen to represent a broad cross-section from the survey. This project has produced a mountain of data which provides the clearest picture so far available of what constitutes a good quality of life in old age. While only a small proportion (50 per cent) rated their quality of life as 'so good it could not be better', around three out of four said that it was good or very good. The chapter highlights the main themes that emerged as the foundations for a good quality of life in old age. Then their very extensive qualitative data, derived from the 80 follow-up interviews, is used to illustrate each of the key themes. These individual descriptions were checked for consistency with the full survey, their own responses to open-ended questions in the survey and regression analyses of the survey data. The central elements of quality in later life that were emphasised consistently by all three methods were: social relationships, home and neighbourhood, psychological well-being and outlook, activities and hobbies (carried out alone), health and functional ability and social roles and activities. Additional key factors were financial circumstances and independence.

Chapter 3 focuses on ethnic minority ageing. James Nazroo and his colleagues report on their use of the concept of quality of life to understand how inequality impacts on the well-being of older ethnic minority people (Bangladeshi, Pakistani, Caribbean and Indian). Their quantitative analysis reveals quality of life variations among ethnic minority groups as well as between them and their white peers and, therefore, suggests a more complex picture than double or triple jeopardy. Independent assessments of economic position, area deprivation and subjective health show a hierarchy of disadvantage ranging from Bangladeshi and Pakistani people at the bottom, through Caribbean and Indian, to white people at the top. Yet subjective assessments of material circumstances, such as crime and community participation, do not show a clear advantage for white people. The chapter also draws on qualitative data to explore more deeply into ethnic inequalities in quality of life. Surprisingly there was a great deal of consistency in the factors identified by respondents as bringing quality to their lives across all four of the ethnic minority groups; although the way these factors featured in people's lives varied by ethnicity. Nazroo and colleagues discuss one specific factor, having a role, and look at paid work, roles in the community and roles as parents and grandparents. As they note, there are inequalities reflecting the disadvantage associated with ethnicity but not uniquely so: both older ethnic minority and white people suffer reduced quality of life because of health and financial problems.

Chapter 4, by Leonie Kellaher, Sheila Peace and Caroline Holland, puts the spotlight on the role in quality of life of the environments in which older people live. They argue rightly that the material and social environment grounds everyday living and set out to understand the dynamic that connects environment to identity and quality of life. They did so by looking at how it operates in a wide variety of living environments and neighbourhoods. Importantly they downgrade previously rigid formulations of quality of life in favour of the dynamic strategies that older people bring into play to enhance the quality of their lives, or to make a 'life of quality'. Using their very rich data they reveal a higher and more complex engagement with the physical and social world by older people than was thought previously to be the case. The life of more or less quality depends on the nature and intensity of the connections a person has with the physical and material environment and the level they want and can manage. In practice older people are constantly generating, reinforcing and dissolving connections with the environment and their range and intensity varies across the lifecourse.

Chapter 5 looks at the quality of life of older people living in England's most deprived urban neighbourhoods. Thomas Scharf, Chris Phillipson and Allison Smith undertook a major field study to investigate the impact of social exclusion on older people living in those areas. Importantly they adapted the multidimensional concept of social exclusion to reflect older people's lives and were able to collect substantial data on the five main dimensions of exclusion: material resources, social relations, civic activities, basic services and neighbourhood. They found that older people in deprived urban areas experience different levels and types of exclusion, with exclusion from social relations being the most common. Moreover a significant proportion (around two-fifths) experienced multiple exclusion and these older people were most likely to be over the age of 75 and from particular ethnic minorities (Pakistani and Somali). This research also demonstrates a clear connection between social exclusion and quality of life.

The sixth chapter by Christina Victor and her colleagues reports on their major investigation into loneliness in old age – the first for 50 years. Echoing the key theme of participation in Chapter 5, this chapter emphasises the importance of social engagement to the quality of older people's lives. The authors compare the results of their quantitative research with those studies carried out in the middle of the last century and find a remarkable degree of consistency in the proportions of older people rating themselves as always or often lonely, but variations in the groups reporting that they are lonely sometimes (increase) or never (decrease). Qualitative research is used to explore older people's experiences and understanding of loneliness and how it might be ameliorated and, specifically, Victor and her colleagues outline three definitions of loneliness and three distinct pathways into loneliness. In terms of ameliorating or preventing loneliness, the main influences identified by older people themselves were family and friends followed by community activities. Factors that 'protect' against loneliness are advanced age and educational qualifications. As well as reporting the key findings from their path-breaking investigation, the authors provide a comprehensive summary of previous research on the vital topic of loneliness in later life.

Chapter 7, by Kate Davidson and Sara Arber, focuses on the health and partnership status of older men. As they say, too little attention has been given to the meanings of health risk to older men and how these are influenced in comparison with the pathological aspects of causality. Their quantitative data analyses revealed a relationship between health and partnership status: lone men were more likely to report poor health than partnered men and married men report the best health (except for those aged 75 and over). Their divorced older men had the poorest health and also the greatest prevalence of health risk behaviours (smoking and alcohol consumption). The qualitative data analysis found a complex picture of health awareness, protection strategies and risk taking. Putting together these two sets of analyses, the authors argue that ideas of independence and masculinity in health matters among younger generations of men persist into later life and continue to influence decisions about seeking professional health care. Nonetheless partnered men are more likely than lone men to seek such advice and take subsequent action.

Chapter 8 by Joanne Cook, Tony Maltby and Lorna Warren reports their innovative study of participation and empowerment as sources of quality in older women's lives. Their research focused on initiatives within the city of Sheffield aimed at including older people and giving them a voice in local policy processes. As the authors point out, at the heart of their research was a participative research approach which attempted to create a real partnership between themselves and the older women 'participants'. This approach generated qualitative data rich in experiences and needs. For many older people involved in this research it was their first opportunity for collective discussion of such matters. The authors show how, when given the right support and opportunity, older women are well able to define and express their own needs and have a strong desire to get their voices heard. Those from ethnic minority groups were keen to see recognition of the needs of their whole community. In this research the participants felt that the route to a better quality of life lay in them being able to voice their own needs and for these to be taken on board in policy and practice. However they faced barriers, such as ageism, racism and language, and consequently felt excluded from services.

The topic of social support among ethnic minority elders is the focus of Chapter 9. Jabeer Butt and Jo Moriarty ground their chapter in the literature on social support and ethnicity. Their research found that, regardless of ethnicity or gender, the vast majority of people were in regular contact with family and friends. Around one-third of them identified family relationships as important in making their life good. The authors describe in detail the types and sources of social support received from families, friends and health and social care services and the levels of satisfaction with and expectations about such support. In a sample in which self-reported health tended to be poor and household incomes comparatively low, it is striking that levels of social support were high. Like the study by Cook and colleagues (Chapter 8) this research revealed the extent to which individuals themselves can influence their social support or be assisted to do so. Like the research by Nazroo and colleagues (Chapter 3), this research emphasises differences between and within black and ethnic minority groups.

In Chapter 10 Lynda Clarke and Ceridwen Roberts report the results of their major investigation into the contribution of grandparenting to quality of life. Their study was based on a representative survey of 870 grandparents of all ages and follow-up interviews with a diverse group of 45 grandparents. Levels of contact were unexpectedly high: three in five grandparents saw at least one grandchild or a set of them on a weekly basis, with proximity being a predictably important determinant of contact. The authors show the critical role of grandparenthood to quality of life: 90 per cent of grandparents under 60 and 85 per cent over 60 said that this was the most important or one of the most important relationships in their life. They draw extensively on their qualitative data to illustrate the felt meaning of grandparenthood which, with a small number of exceptions, was wholly positive.

Chapter 11 concentrates on the quality of the lives of frail older people living in residential institutions; those referred to in Chapter 8 as having 'quiet voices'. As Susan Tester and her colleagues point out, this group has rarely been the focus of quality of life research and those for whom communication is difficult have been largely excluded from research (Farquhar 1995; Walker and Walker 1998). The team made great efforts to communicate with frail older people, including those with dementia. Contrary to the popular tendency to homogenise older people and especially those in institutions, this research emphasises the individuality of frail older people. They demonstrate, for the first time, the importance of communication for quality of life, even if this is non-verbal. They highlight the key positive impacts on quality of life, such as the older person's strengths in response to frailty and being able to assert control and rights; as well as the key negative ones such as negative responses to the person's frailty and dependence and loss of control and being controlled. This chapter is rounded off by some practical proposals aimed at promoting good quality of life in institutional care.

In the concluding chapter Catherine Hagan Hennessy mentions the key cross-cutting themes that not only run through the ten projects represented in this book but the programme as a whole. The four themes emphasised – the meaning given to quality of life by older people, and the influences on quality of life of the environments in which people live, social participation and ethnicity – are of major importance in both understanding quality of life in old age and for the development of policies to enhance quality of life. These themes will be elaborated in the companion volume to this one. Chapter 12 concludes with a look forward to a new interdisciplinary research programme that will pick up these key themes, as well as others arising from the GO Programme, and subject them to analysis from the perspective of different disciplines.

I am certain that I represent all of the authors of this book and, indeed, everyone associated with the GO Programme, when I hope that the wealth of scientific evidence contained here and in the subsequent volumes will not only be of great benefit to students and researchers in helping to understand quality of life in old age and to develop even more sophisticated ways of enabling older people to articulate their needs, but will also inform policy and practice so that more older people can live lives of quality.

Box 1.1　ESRC Growing Older Programme projects

Project title	Project leader
How older people sustain their identities and preferences in the face of a limiting physical condition and the need to accept health and care services	John Baldock
Quality of life of the healthy elderly: residential setting and social comparison processes	Graham Beaumont
Adding quality to quantity. Older people's views on their quality of life and its enhancement	Ann Bowling
Spiritual beliefs and existential meaning in later life: the experience of older bereaved spouses	Peter Coleman
An anthropological investigation of lay and professional meanings of quality of life	Christopher McKevitt
Environment and identity in later life: a cross-setting study	Sheila M. Peace
Influences on quality of life in early old age	David Blane
Inequalities in quality of life among people aged 75 and over and in the community	Elizabeth Breeze
Ethnic inequalities in quality of life at older ages: subjective and objective components	James Nazroo

Older people in deprived neighbourhoods: social exclusion and quality of life in old age	Thomas Scharf
Exploring perceptions of quality of life of frail older people during and after the transition to institutional care	Susan Tester
Quality of life and real life cognitive functioning	Mary Gilhooly
Transport and ageing – extending quality of life for older people via public and private transport	Mary Gilhooly
Evaluating the impact of reminiscence on quality of life of older people	Kevin McKee
Older people's experience of paid employment: participation and quality of life	Ivan Robertson
Older men: their social world and healthy lifestyles	Sara Arber
Older widow(er)s: bereavement and gender effects on lifestyle and participation	Kate Bennett
Family, work and quality of life: changing economic and social roles	Maria Evandrou
Quality of life and social support among older people from different ethnic groups	Jabeer Butt
Grandparenthood: its meaning and its contribution to older people's quality of life	Lynda Clarke
Older women's lives and voices: participation and policy in Sheffield	Lorna Warren
Older people and lifelong learning: choices and experiences	Alexandra Withnall
Empowerment and disempowerment: comparative study of Afro-Caribbean, Asian and White British women in their third age.	Mary Maynard
Loneliness, social isolation and living alone in later life	Christina Victor

2

Quality of Life in Old Age from the Perspectives of Older People

Zahava Gabriel and Ann Bowling

Introduction

The literature on quality of life (QoL) suggests that it reflects both macro societal and socio-demographic influences on people as well as the characteristics and concerns of individuals. Thus, it could be argued that societies overall hold a common core of values, and their presence or absence influences macro societal QoL. However, as QoL is also subjective, it is equally dependent upon the interpretations and perceptions of the individual (Ziller 1974). As such, the definition and measurement of QoL should be grounded empirically both in lay views and reflect the concept's individual subjectivity and variation, while at the same time taking account of wider social circumstances. Unfortunately, traditional models of QoL are rarely multi-level or multi-domain. They range from basic, objective and subjective needs-based approaches derived from Maslow's (1954) hierarchy of human needs, to classic models based on psychological well-being, happiness, morale and life satisfaction (Andrews 1986; Andrews and Withey 1976; Larson 1978), physical health and functioning (see Bowling 2001 for examples), social expectations models (Calman 1983) and models based on the individual's unique perceptions (O'Boyle 1997). Social gerontologists also focus on the importance of social and personal resources, self-mastery or control over life, autonomy (freedom to determine one's own actions or behaviour) and independence (the ability to act on one's own or for oneself, without being controlled or dependent on anything or anyone else for one's functioning) (Baltes and Baltes 1990). Due to an increasing acknowledgement of the multifaceted nature of QoL, researchers now often base their model of QoL on combinations of these domains, for example, the World Health Organization's WHOQOL Group model (WHQOL Group 1993).

While social gerontologists in the United States have a long tradition of investigating life satisfaction, correlates of 'the good life' and positive as well as negative aspects of ageing (Andrews 1986), in Europe, a main body of social research has been heavily influenced by the positivist perspective of functionalism and focused on decline and disability. In much of Europe this has led to a negative focus on ageing as a time of dependency, poverty, service need, and declining physical and mental health. The care needs of dependent older people have been emphasised at the expense of rehabilitation, prevention and curative treatment once medical problems have been detected (Roos and Havens 1991). Research based on this model has inevitably underestimated the QoL of older people. Gradual realisation of the flaws in this focus has shifted the emphasis towards a more positive view of old age as a natural component of the life span (O'Boyle 1997), which can provide personal fulfilment.

At the individual level, existing models of QoL in older age can find some support in research on older people's perceptions of it (Farquhar 1995; Fry 2000; Bowling et al. 2002). However, research which has tapped lay views is limited. The implication is that most existing models of QoL have not been grounded in older people's views and priorities, and thus have not been tested adequately for content validity. How people construct their QoL at various levels also remains a neglected area of research which is an increasingly important area for research and public policy.

This chapter reports the results of a national survey on QoL and qualitative follow-up interviews with a subsample of survey respondents. It draws on interview data from 999 people aged 65 and over living at home in Britain which asked older people about the quality of their lives and how that quality can be improved. The survey data (analysis of open-ended responses and regression models) is referred to more briefly here as a point of comparison and to provide wider context for the qualitative data, and has been published elsewhere (Bowling et al. 2002; Bowling et al. 2004; Bowling and Gabriel 2004).

Aims and methods

The aim of the analyses presented here was to contribute to the development of a conceptual framework and body of knowledge on QoL in older age, grounded in older people's views. The Quality of Life Survey aimed to identify all respondents aged 65 and over living at home to the four quarterly Office for National Statistics (ONS) Omnibus Surveys in Britain and to include them in the Quality of Life Survey. All respondents aged 65 and over who were interviewed for the Omnibus Survey (April, September, November, 2000, January 2001 surveys) were asked at the end of that interview if they would be willing to be reinterviewed by ONS interviewers for our module on Quality of Life. Those who consented to participate further were reinterviewed for the Quality of Life Survey two months after their Omnibus Survey interview.

The Quality of Life Survey interviews were conducted with a sample (999) of 1299 eligible respondents from the Omnibus Survey sample respondents aged 65+. The interviews were carried out in their own homes. Full details of the method and sample have been published elsewhere (Bowling et al. 2004). Further in-depth interviews about QoL were carried out 12 to 18 months later with a subsample of 80 of the 999 participants in the Quality of Life Survey based on respondents' socio-demographic characteristics and health status, QoL ratings and region of residence. The aim was to interview a broad cross-section of respondents to the survey in order to obtain a better understanding of people's interpretations of QoL. One year later, brief telephone interviews elicited changes in the lives of half of this group of respondents and they were subsequently reinterviewed in depth to explore these further.

Characteristics of the survey respondents and those who were subsequently followed up in depth

The socio-demographic characteristics of respondents to the Quality of Life Survey, who were all interviewed during 2000 and early 2001, were similar in their distributions to people aged 65+ in Britain, compared with mid-term population estimates from the 1991 Census, and compared with respondents aged 65+ living at home in the comparable General Household Survey (GHS) and other national surveys

(Bridgwood et al. 2000; Walker et al. 2001; Falaschetti et al. 2002). About half, 48 per cent (480), of the Quality of Life Survey respondents were female and 52 per cent (519) were male. Of the QoL survey respondents, 62 per cent (624) were aged 65 to 74 and 38 per cent (375) were aged 75+; the comparable figures for the GHS in 2000 were 58 per cent and 42 per cent respectively. The comparable figures for respondents aged 65+ to the GHS in 2000 were 51 per cent female and 49 per cent male (2000). Ninety-eight per cent (983) of QoL respondents were white, again as would be expected from national statistics.

The in-depth follow-up sample taken from the respondents to the survey included 40 men and 40 women, ranging in age from 65 to 69 to over 80; half were married and the remainder were single, widowed, separated or divorced; 36 had an income of less than £6240 per annum and the rest had more than this. They represented six widely spread regions of England and Scotland.

Findings

The 999 survey respondents were asked to rate their overall QoL on a 7-point Likert scale from 'So good it could not be better' to 'So bad it could not be worse'. There were no statistically significant differences with overall QoL ratings ('good', 'bad' or 'most important') and age or gender. For example, 4 per cent (21) of males and 6 per cent (32) of females rated their QoL as 'So good it could not be better', 78 per cent (404) and 70 per cent (362) of males and females respectively labelled it as 'Very good' or 'Good' and the remainder rated it from 'Alright' to 'So bad it could not be worse'. There were no consistent seasonal effects with QoL ratings.

A model of QoL emerged from respondents' descriptions of the quality of their lives. The themes forming the foundations for a good QoL which emerged from both the open-ended survey responses and the in-depth follow-up interviews overlapped considerably (Bowling and Gabriel 2004). The main themes were:

+ good social relationships with family, friends and neighbours

+ good home and neighbourhood (safe, good facilities including transport)

+ positive outlook and psychological well-being

- activities/hobbies (performed alone)

- good health and functional ability

- social roles and engaging in social and voluntary activities (with others)

- adequate income

- independence and control over one's life.

Table 2.1 Older people's definitions of the constituents of QoL (in-depth interviews)

Constituent	Good things that give their life quality		Bad things that take quality away from their lives		Mentioned good or bad	
	% resp.	(n)*	% resp.	(n)*	% resp.	(n)*
Social relationships	96	(77)	80	(64)	99	(79)
Home and neighbourhood	96	(77)	84	(67)	100	(80)
Psychological well-being	96	(77)	63	(50)	99	(79)
Other activities done alone	93	(74)	–	(0)	93	(74)
Health	85	(68)	83	(66)	99	(79)
Social roles and activities	80	(64)	1	(1)	80	(64)
Financial circumstances	73	(58)	53	(42)	91	(73)
Independence	69	(55)	46	(37)	84	(67)
Other/miscellaneous	18	(14)	19	(15)	31	(25)
Society/politics	1	(1)	43	(34)	43	(34)
Number of respondents	**80**		**80**		**80**	

Note: Includes heterogeneous subgroups: good only, bad only, good or bad themes mentioned (single counting only). Reproduced with permission from Baywood Publishing Company (*International Journal of Aging and Human Development*).

These are shown for the in-depth interviews in Table 2.1. Multiple regression models were conducted on the main survey data (Bowling et al. 2002) for the 999 respondents, based on their responses to structured measurement scales, with QoL rating as the dependent variable. These showed that the main independent predictors, or drivers, of self-rated QoL in older age, which predicted over 25 per cent of the variance in QoL ratings (Adjusted R^2) were:

* people's standards of social comparison and expectations in life

* a sense of optimism and belief that 'all will be well in the end' rather than a tendency to think the worst (or glass 'half full' rather than 'half empty' perspective on life)

* having good health and physical functioning

* engaging in a large number of social activities and feeling supported

* living in a neighbourhood with good community facilities and services, including transport, feeling safe in one's neighbourhood.

These themes were consistent with the themes that emerged from the semi-structured and unstructured approaches, although income and control over life (a measure of independence) did not retain statistical significance in the models.

Examples of the overall themes mentioned from the in-depth interviews with the 80 follow-up respondents provide insight into why the domains of QoL highlighted in this study were important to people. More detailed categorisation of the themes is available from the authors (see www.shef.ac.uk/uni/projects/gop/).

Social relationships with family, friends and neighbours

Table 2.1 illustrates that having good social resources was cited as part of having a good QoL by almost all respondents. Regular face-to-face contact with families was said to be important to having a good QoL by 59 respondents out of 80 (74 per cent). Sixty-two per cent (50 people) said they had 'good relationships' with relatives (that is emotionally supportive and loving relationships). These were the type of relationships which enabled respondents to feel that others cared about them and would always be there for them if they had a problem.

Some people, particularly those who were widowed, appreciated the company and emotional support which their children or other relatives provided. Others spoke of the importance of knowing that there is someone to call on if they have a problem, particularly if their children were living nearby. Some respondents simply enjoyed spending time with their families and seeing them living happy lives:

Interviewer (I):   And what would be the good things giving your life quality?

Respondent (R):   Being near my family ... they come when we need them, and they're all very good to us ... we're very close to each other, I think that's really good.

I: And how often do you see your family?

R: We either go to them, or [they] come to us, and we're old and doddery now ... or they think we are ... we see one or other of them most weekends, and ... if not, we go to them, they invite us to lunch, or something like that. So, we have a good life, really.

Forty-five per cent (36 respondents) said their QoL was enhanced through contact with their grandchildren, because it gave them an emotional boost to spend time with children and teenagers. Respondents also enjoyed a reciprocal relationship with their grandchildren. They liked to give advice and spoil their grandchildren while they gained pleasure from seeing them happy and feeling loved by them. Some people enjoyed holidays with their grandchildren and others liked to have their grandchildren staying at their homes. They also appreciated the practical help which older grandchildren could provide.

Forty-six per cent (37) also said they enjoyed seeing friends for company and the opportunity to do things with others (particularly if they were widowed). However, they also said they appreciated the emotional support and close contact which good friends provided.

Not all relationships were said to be good. Twenty-nine per cent (23) said they worried about or felt responsible for, members of their family and this detracted from their QoL. Worries included younger family members' finances, poor health and relationship problems, such as adult children's marital break-ups. In some cases, respondents still felt responsible for their adult children as well as their grandchildren and would either support them financially and/or by minding their grandchildren. Some people also felt responsible for very elderly relatives. They either spoke of caring for ageing relatives in poor health or having to cope with their deaths by taking on an organisational role, such as arranging funerals:

It's a responsibility of sons, daughters, nieces and nephews – whichever way you look at it ... to care for ... the senior family ... I mean, my aunt's house, which we cleared ... she died suddenly, and we estimate it took us some 400 hours to go through the house. We were going down on Friday nights ... and coming back exhausted on Sundays, having had to go through absolutely everything.

Seventeen deaths in the last five years ... in the extended family ... our responsibilities in that ... are now over thank goodness – but we had frail relatives in homes or in care of one form or another ... we have had to do the round of homes, power of attorney, and all the rest of it, and of course that puts a drain on your finances, because you ... you pay your own fare to go and visit them. Invariably it's a night's accommodation for two, and what do you do when you get there? You don't want to sit in the lounge with other people who are nodding off ... they sit there all week, or all ... month or whatever since you last saw them, so you put them in the car, and take them out to lunch ... And then, of course, you'd take him somewhere, maybe walk him to a seat and sit on the prom for an hour, or put him in the wheelchair ... cup of tea, back in the car, back to where they ... came from. Sort the bills out, and ... drive home again.

Twenty-two per cent (18) mentioned losses which detracted from quality in their lives, including missing friends who had died or moved away from the neighbourhood and ten respondents mentioned missing family members who had died. This was said to have a great effect on their QoL, often leading to loneliness. They also missed spending time with their friends or relatives, speaking on the phone with them and gaining advice from confidants.

Seventeen per cent (14) said that they did not see their family as much as they would like to and 20 per cent (16) spoke of their children and grandchildren being 'too busy' to see them. This was sometimes used as a justification to help older people to feel better about not seeing their children and grandchildren regularly:

I'd like to see me son ... Our son doesn't get home till about half past seven. We were down there Sunday ... But of course he's got his family, and the boy plays football, and he takes him to football and takes him training on Saturday, and his wife works on Sunday. And so ... his time's taken up.

Underlying the value placed on social relationships, then, was the prevention of loneliness, provision of company and entertainment, the need for reciprocal emotional support, feeling cared for, maintaining confidence, having someone to talk to, to provide advice, to call on for everyday help and in emergencies.

Home and neighbourhood

Neighbourhood resources or neighbourhood social capital were also said to contribute to good QoL by a majority of respondents. Sixty-one per cent (49) indicated that having good relationships with their neighbours contributed to good QoL. In place of having family living nearby, neighbours could take on the role of providing security. This involved the reassurance that there was always someone looking out for them and someone who would provide help if it was needed. Relationships with neighbours involving the exchange of practical help such as lifts to the doctor and help with shopping were also highly valued. People spoke positively about having an age mix within the neighbourhood.

For some respondents, neighbours were also regarded as friends with whom they spent a lot of time. Close relationships with neighbours are likely to be important for older people when they may lack the transport or physical mobility required to visit friends living further away, or when they are ill:

> My neighbours are very good. Them over there could be called at any-time in emergency at any time. He watch me through my toilet window. If my toilet window is open, I'm out. ... my neighbour takes me to Sainsbury's every Tuesday, but Wednesday this week. But ... he always takes me for the last three years, so I think that's very good of him.

During their interviews two-fifths (33) mentioned that enjoyment of the area in which they lived enhanced their QoL. They said they enjoyed pleasant views and areas in which to take 'nice walks' as well as the sense of belonging to a community. Good facilities and local services were also important (shops, markets, post office, health services, street lighting, refuse collection, police, local mobile/library). Just over one-third (28) also mentioned deriving pleasure from their own homes and stated that this contributed to their QoL. In some cases, they felt proud of having lived in their homes for many years and associated their homes with happy memories of the past, for example, bringing up their children:

> I love my house ... Well I've been here 23 years ... and I've got the most wonderful view as you can from this window ... It's beautiful, and from my bedroom window ... I can see X ... oh yes, I should miss all that ... Imagine just sat there ... and looking into somebody else's window across the road ... And just seeing traffic going up and down ... that doesn't appeal to me at all. I think I've got a good quality of life for myself ... I mean there's others, I mean their health is against them for one thing, and probably where they're living is another.

Good public transport was said to contribute to QoL of 38 per cent (31). They appreciated free bus passes or discount fares for older people, so that they could travel without worrying about being able to afford to reach certain places. Having comfortable buses and a regular and reliable service was also important. In addition, buses with a drop step, making it easier to get on and off, were valued:

> I think that the fact that they gave us a free pass, which means that you can [travel], if you haven't got money, I've got money that through my husband working ... I can do it but so many people that I do meet on the buses have their passes; that is the most wonderful thing, I think that is one of the things this country's done that's helped people, and I think that they should do it even more, in more places, cause my sister lives in W and she didn't have that help ... But I mean it's made it wonderful for people round here because you can go up to B on the bus free ... buses is the most important thing to me.

Poor public transport was said to have a negative impact on the QoL of 32 per cent (26). Some of these people said that it was more difficult to get out and about because of inadequate transport and uncomfortable buses could be painful for respondents with joint or mobility problems. Similarly, walking to distant bus stops (particularly in inclement weather or on icy streets in the winter) and getting on and off the older style buses, which lacked drop steps could be difficult for them. Financial constraints could also reduce people's use of public transport. Even with discounted bus fares for retired people, some respondents spoke of expensive fares for short distances, which they could not afford. They also expressed the feeling that after a difficult journey they would not be relaxed enough to enjoy themselves:

> So ... you don't go nowhere. And I sit here at the top of this hill, in this flat, belonging to B2 council ... I live here, there's just one [bus route], and if it doesn't want to run, it doesn't ... And there's not just me on this road, there's more elderly ... So you've got to walk up the hill because there's nothing to bring you, because the bus isn't there. And if it's winter, and it's icy, well you stay in, darling. That's when you rely on your children ... But the bus fares are atrocious. I mean it's nearly a pound, to go up – so that's taking two pound, if you go there and come back, that's two pound ... Not everybody's got two pound to spare, love ... so it's all wrong.

Poor local services and facilities more generally were said to adversely affect the QoL of 26 per cent (21). Some of these individuals felt that they were not given enough information about the facilities and activities available for older people in their area. Others claimed that there was inadequate provision of social activities for older people run by their local council. They wanted to see educational and exercise classes that were close enough for them to attend. Some also expressed concern over the lack of a local police presence. Just over one-fifth (17) stated that they felt unsafe and some also spoke positively about former times when they felt safer. For those in poor health the state of the roads in their local area was important in order to prevent uncomfortable and painful journeys by bus and car.

Thus, underlying the value placed on home and neighbourhood were having good neighbours who could provide friendship, be alert for emergencies, provide help and support if frail or ill, and substitute for relatives. Also valued were having a pleasant environment to live in, a community spirit, and having good local facilities, leisure activities, feeling safe, and having accessible, affordable public transport.

Psychological well-being and outlook

People's lives and actions are influenced by their mental outlook, attitudes and personality characteristics. Almost all respondents stated that their own personalities and experiences contributed to their overall QoL. This often involved personal philosophies about life and the way in which events and circumstances were interpreted by them (for example, with an optimistic or pessimistic perspective). The positive influences on QoL that were mentioned included having a positive attitude rather than feeling sorry for themselves or worrying about life, in particular a content and/or even-tempered disposition (mentioned by 57 per cent), an optimistic approach to life, and being able to look forward to things (mentioned by 16 per cent).

Others spoke about 'taking each day as it comes' and not worrying about what might happen in the future. Some also mentioned the importance of acceptance and 'making the best of things' (that is making the best of what they do have, rather than focusing on the negative parts of their lives), which had sometimes developed from their upbringing and earlier experiences (for example, wartime childhoods).

Coping strategies of acceptance of one's lot were employed by 47 per cent (38) to help them face the negative changes of ageing, such as losing health and mobility and bereavement:

> I think acceptance – I've found when I've had, like when my first husband was killed in a road accident, and my second husband, he sat and died suddenly ... you've got to accept that these things have happened, and you've got to move on. I think so anyway ... I mean there's some people ... oh, she'll never get over that, well you never do get over it but if you can accept it you can start taking the steps, you've got to ... life's got to go on, hasn't it? ... I think acceptance and contentment, they're the sort of things ... That's my simple philosophy. But I've lived by it ... and I've got where I am ... but as I say ... if some pensioners had £500 a week they still wouldn't be satisfied, they'd want six, wouldn't they?

Two-fifths (32) spoke of making a conscious effort to keep busy in order to prevent despondency. They viewed a good QoL as an active and varied life. They wanted to continue to take on all that life offered them as much as they could, in spite of the negative changes they associated with older age, such as having less energy and poorer health. Respondents did not let themselves watch TV during the day, so that they did not waste whole days in front of the television. Others completed a daily crossword or memorised facts or poems in order to remain mentally active and prevent dementia. The most explicit expression of these ideas was from two people who claimed that people make their own QoL. In the words of one of them:

Quality of life is what you make it, you can't buy it, or inherit it, or anything like that, you know. So ... as I say, it's what you make it.

Many people said that negative feelings detracted from their QoL. For example, three out of ten (25) mentioned negative feelings about the future. Such fears were strongly linked to ageing and involved worries about losing health and/or independence:

I mean I often think well, what is there to look forward to, in old age ... it can be frightening if you think about it, you think of all these people and friends of course that have been ill or are ill or have died and you think 'oh, is this what's going to happen to us?' ... the thing which would frighten me the most would be going in a home.

Twelve per cent (10) reported their QoL as being affected negatively by the past. Bad memories of the past could affect their QoL, and in some cases respondents felt that autobiographical events had shaped their current QoL. One-tenth (8) also reported having periods of depression and/or were unhappy with their lives, which adversely affected their QoL. Most of these people with poor well-being reported that they had suffered from negative life events and circumstances, for example, deaths of partners, other family members and/or friends. The multiple adverse life events that can accompany older age, especially loss of family and friends through death, can have a major impact on psychological well-being and mental health (for example, depression).

Respondents often commented on the multifaceted nature of QoL, and the interdependency of its components. Thus poor psychological well-being and outlook were sometimes due to the experience of adverse life events, for example, bereavements and their memories, fears of ageing, ill health and dependency, and the future. Conversely, respondents who also emphasised having a good outlook on life, which contributed to a good QoL, stressed the importance of being optimistic in life, looking forward to things, being thankful for (still) being alive, being content, trying to enjoy life, being open to new activities, keeping busy, acceptance of situations and downward adjustment of expectations, as well as making downward social comparisons with others who were worse off in order to maintain positive well-being, and making the best of things. Respondents with these perspectives tended to feel one made one's own (good) QoL.

Social activities and hobbies (communal and solo)

Some people mentioned the importance of 'keeping busy' in relation to psychological well-being. This also emerged when most of them raised the value of social activities to their QoL, including reciprocal activities such as voluntary work and helping other people, which made them feel valued. Undertaking voluntary work was said to contribute to having a good QoL by 21 per cent (17) and for some was one way of keeping busy and remaining active after retirement:

> I want to keep active, I want to contribute to society, and I've been very fortunate in what society's given me, as it were, in successful, professional – and one wants to give something back ... So that's what I've done.

Engaging in activities which were mentally stimulating was said to be important for the QoL of 21 per cent (17). Some people perceived older age as a time for learning new skills which they did not have the chance to learn previously. Attending educational classes, for example, enabled respondents to meet new people and served as a regular forum for socialising, as well as stimulating their minds.

Going on holiday or for weekends away was also important for 45 per cent (36) as they enjoyed seeing new places, getting some sun and relaxing. They also appreciated having a break from their routine and responsibilities at home. For example, Mrs O, who had been caring for her ill aunt and often looked after her grandchildren, described how much she had enjoyed going away by herself for the first time:

> When you've had a long run looking after people, you feel like a relaxed break, so ... last year ... I wanted to get away on my own, and I've never done it in my life ... and I had a gorgeous time ... I went to ... Scotland, with B, our coach people ... it really did me good to get away from ... everyone I knew, and everything that I normally do ... So I've booked a holiday this year again in August ... I'm going to the Isle of Wight ... I think you need to, sometimes, just get that break.

Thus, the pursuit of social activities was important to people for retaining an interest in life, keeping busy and active, and for meeting other people. Some activities, including those done alone, were valued because they provided mental stimulation, which people saw as important for their mental health. Voluntary work was valued for its reciprocal nature, and people liked to feel both valued and that they were giving something back to society in their retirement.

Health

Most people said that having good health was critical to a good QoL and this was sometimes related to their expectations of poorer health in older age. Some referred to being able to do what they wanted to as a result of having good health:

> I suppose health's the main thing, cause you've got no quality of life if you haven't got your health, have you?

> I think that number 1 is having good health ... Because without that you are restricted ... I mean the other things follow on, like being able to go to the gym which I have just done, swim, we play bridge a lot.

Similarly, a large proportion also reported that deteriorating health adversely affected their QoL. Two-fifths (32) mentioned not being fit enough to do what they want to do, and having to give up activities, including driving, because of their poor health. Respondents frequently said they coped with their health-related problems by accepting them.

The poor health of close others was said to have had a considerable impact on the QoL of just over one-quarter (21). This was due to worry about a spouse's or another close relative's health, or the burden of providing care which can be most traumatic in the case of someone with Alzheimer's:

> My quality of life is overwhelmingly ... altered, and focused by my wife's ... problems ... I've often thought. I look after three people. My wife used to look after me, she used to feed me, she used to do my laundry ... If I was ill she'd nurse me ... She'd make sure my tie was on straight ... that kind of thing, and now I have to do all that for myself. I do everything for her; she does nothing. I do the washing up, the laundry, the ironing, the dusting ... the vacuum cleaning, all the financial stuff, she doesn't know what money is ... so I look after two people, really I didn't look after anyone before. I did my job ... I didn't have to think about who was going to press me trousers or who was going to wash me shirt, I did none of those – well now I do it all, and I do it all for her. And then there is a third person, a third person undoes all I do, the third person hides me keys, the third person floods the kitchen by leaving the

taps on in the bathroom, the third person hides my letters ... it's all stress and strain. And of course that very much affects my quality of life.

Deteriorating health, their own or a close other's, was mentioned by most respondents as the domain that had changed one year later at their follow-up interview.

Financial circumstances

Many respondents associated having a good QoL with being financially secure or comfortable. They were generally modest in their expectations. They often spoke about the importance of having enough money to pay their bills, not having to worry about money, and knowing that sufficient money was available should an unexpected expense arise. Some said that they appreciated having enough money to do and buy what they wanted:

> It's (QoL) having sufficient money, I mean not excessive money, just enough to do what you require, run your car, say, and pay your bills, and have the odd holiday. I don't mean thousands of pounds or millions of pounds, but sufficient money not to have to worry about money.

These people also linked their finances to their ability to enjoy life (that is being able to afford to do the things they enjoy doing). Some respondents associated enjoyment with QoL while others stressed empowerment. It was an instrument which enabled them to do the things they liked doing. Several people also mentioned feeling lucky about their financial situation, and downwardly compared themselves to others perceived to have less money. Mrs J made downward comparisons between her own financial situation, with the benefit of a private pension, and those of her friends who lived only on a state pension.

> I'm ... fairly fortunate, I've been able to live quite happily and go on holidays and things [laughs] which a lot of old people can't, especially those who only have their state pension – I don't know how they cope, to be honest. ... I know we've had the £5 rise ... But then the council tax goes up, and TV licences go up, everything goes up – £5 really goes nowhere [laughs] but as I say I'm fortunate, I have a work pension, and I have half of my husband's work pension, so, I, I'm not too bad, but, it, ... I do feel sorry for a lot of my friends, I know they really are hard up.

Some people were upset that they could not afford to buy new furniture, or that they could not afford to decorate their homes. Others could not afford sufficient domestic help, which they said they needed because of their declining health and mobility. Eleven per cent (9) living on a state pension felt that they could not afford to enjoy life:

I: And you mentioned not enough money ... what kind of things would you buy...?

R: Well, I'd have a holiday for a start ... a good thing would be to be able to go to the cinema, I can't remember the last time I went there, or, well, or theatrical, or a train ride, or little things that needs money ... Can't do anything on £53 a week ... It's not enough to really enjoy life. I mean it's enough to get through, but what can you do on £53 ... But you know, we all pull together, me and [inaudible] me husband ... we just get through ... but nothing spare ... So, I mean that does affect your life. If you've got money you can move, can't you – even if you're not very good on your legs you can order taxis like you did ... You can't do that on what I get.

Thus money was important to QoL, not just in terms of ensuring that basic needs were met, but in enabling people to participate in society, to enjoy themselves, and to free them from worry about paying bills, not being able to meet emergencies, or paying for practical help when needed.

Independence

Over two-thirds of respondents emphasised the importance of retaining their independence for their QoL. In this context, being able to walk and having good mobility was mentioned by just over a quarter (21) as being important to them. They said they wanted to avoid the boredom and monotony of a life confined indoors through immobility, and wanted to continue to be able to do things for themselves, such as shopping and household tasks. Avoidance of dependency on others was a commonly held value. Retaining their mobility and independence was also said to be important to respondents because it enabled them to get outdoors and continue to enjoy life, and to meet other people.

Sixteen per cent (13) also appreciated the greater independence from time constraints, and ensuing flexibility that they had since retiring, and said that this contributed to a good QoL. Without the pressures of working long hours, commuting to work, or juggling family and work, these respondents felt they had more time to enjoy life, to see their family and friends, and to take up hobbies and new social activities. This also enabled them to 'lie in' bed in the mornings, to stay up late at night, to eat at more varied times, and to take more short breaks away and holidays.

Sixteen per cent (13) described how having a car gave their lives quality, as it meant they did not have to rely on public transport or on lifts from other people and could be independent:

> All we do is shopping, but I mean, I couldn't really put on my husband, because he's had a stroke and two heart attacks, so we couldn't go down the road and carry our shopping home. So we do need transport, although as I say – I have got a son and a daughter that've got cars, but they're working, so ... you can't sort of, put on them all the time, you can't expect them to do everything for you. You've got to be independent as much as possible. Yeah. So I think, without the car, we'd be pretty stuck.

Fourteen per cent (11) who were unable to drive or who did not have access to a car felt that this detracted from their QoL by decreasing their independence. Sometimes, they were reliant on public transport, often with a poor or infrequent service, which prevented them from travelling, seeing people and doing things they would like to do. Some of the women expressed regret at not having learnt to drive, or were prevented from continuing to drive due to poor health. In each case they became dependent on their husbands for lifts. Alternatively, widowed women who were unable to drive missed going out in the car with their husbands and pursuing the activities which this enabled them to do:

> I used to ... play bridge, which I love, but unfortunately ... I can't go out at night, now, you see, because ... I haven't a car ... But ... that would improve my quality of life: to be able to play bridge again.

Seven per cent (6) reported that they lacked energy or were in poor health, which prevented them from being able to do things for themselves. Being unable to do their shopping or housework, or being unable to out for a walk, led to feelings of frustration. Thus the maintenance of independence in older age was important to people. Respondents disliked being dependent on others for help, or even for lifts. Independence was threatened by poor health and impaired mobility, and by lack of access to transport. On the positive side, independence was enhanced in older age when people were freed from the constraints placed on them by working hours. Independence was enhanced if they had retained their health, had an adequate income and access to a car.

Conclusion

This chapter has presented the descriptions of QoL which emerged from in-depth interviews with a sample of 80 respondents to the Quality of Life Survey. Their descriptions were consistent with those of all 999 survey respondents, in their replies to open-ended survey questions, and overlapped with those of the regression model based on the structured survey data.

These findings are unique in that they were empirically grounded in older people's views which were elicited using a triangulated approach. They also highlighted how areas of QoL are interlinked, and have knock-on effects. The results from the triangulated approaches indicated that overall QoL is built on a series of interrelated drivers (main themes). These reflected commonly held core values, while individuals also emphasised constituent subthemes reflecting the variations between their lives. Greater recognition is needed in definitions of QoL research that influencing variables are not only people's own personal characteristics and circumstances, but that there is also a dynamic interplay between people and their surrounding social structures in a changing society.

The central planks of QoL, which were emphasised consistently by all three methods, were social relationships, home and neighbourhood social capital, psychological well-being and outlook, activities and hobbies (solo), health and functional ability and social roles and activities. The lay models also emphasised the importance of financial circumstances and independence, which need to be incorporated into a broader definition of QoL. Moving beyond health and functional status and their impact on life, as a proxy concept and measure for QoL, is important to achieving a better understanding of the quality of later life.

A model of QoL and its measurement scales needs to be based on these concepts. Thus QoL can be said to be about having good social relationships, help and support; living in a home and neighbourhood perceived to give pleasure, and which feels safe, and is neighbourly, with access to local facilities and services, including transport; engaging in hobbies and leisure activities (solo) as well as maintaining social activities and retaining a role in society; having a positive psychological outlook and acceptance of circumstances which cannot be changed; having good health and mobility, having enough money to meet basic needs and to enable people to participate in society and to enjoy life, and to retain one's independence and control over life.

The policy implications of people's views generally focus on enabling older people to maintain their health and independence, social activities, and relationships. Respondents emphasised the importance of living in a neighbourly and safe area, and having good local facilities to promote friendly and helpful relationship with other people, including neighbours. This was also seen to be important in preventing loneliness and isolation. The availability of good local facilities was also seen as important. Creation of local opportunities to meet other people and to maintain a role in society (for example, work or voluntary work), access to transport and having enough money were necessary for retaining independence. The results also indicate that: people should be encouraged to develop positive thinking and direct their perceptions upwards; they need to learn to be, and to feel, more in control of their everyday lives and its competing demands; these characteristics are likely to enhance their coping skills in the face of the challenges of older age. Dubos (1959) observed that the goals which people set for themselves and the way in which they adapt to them are as responsible for health and ill health as diseases and other external challenges.

People also need to involve themselves in social activities and build up their support networks from young age onwards. The importance of health and functioning underlines yet again the need to adopt healthy lifestyles and preventive health strategies throughout life in order to help retain independence. In addition, society needs to work harder, and in partnership with local people, to promote local communities with good facilities, opportunities for social participation, increased independence, affordable and accessible transport and services, and environments which are perceived to be safe. Society also has a collective responsibility to ensure that retirement pensions are adequate in order to enable people to experience a good QoL in older age.

Acknowledgements

We are grateful to ONS Omnibus Survey staff and the ONS Qualitative Research Unit, in particular Olga Evans, Maureen Kelly, Olwen Rowlands, Jack Eldridge and Kirsty Deacon for their much appreciated advice and help with designing the questionnaire, for conducting focus groups with older people to inform the questionnaire design, for sampling and overseeing the Quality of Life Interview and processing the data. We are also grateful to Matthew Bond for advice with statistical analysis, Anne Fleissig and Lee Marriott-Dowding for assistance with the open coding and the development of the coding frames, ONS interviewers and to the respondents themselves.

Those who carried out the original analysis and collection of the data hold no responsibility for its further analysis and interpretation. Material from the ONS Omnibus Survey, made available through ONS, has been used with the permission of the Controller of The Stationery Office. The dataset will be held on the Data Archive at the University of Essex. The research was funded by the Economic and Social Research Council (award no. L480254003 – Quality of Life). The Quality of Life Questionnaire was also part-funded by grants, held collaboratively, by Professor Christina Victor and Professor John Bond (L480254042; Loneliness and Social Isolation, also part of the ESRC Growing Older Research Programme) and by Professor Shah Ebrahim (Medical Research Council Health Services Research Collaboration – Health and Disability). The authors are grateful for their support.

3

Ethnic inequalities

James Nazroo, Madhavi Bajekal, David Blane and Ini Grewal

Introduction

The ethnic make-up of the UK population and how this has changed has been well documented (Barot 1996; Modood et al. 1997; Mason 2003), especially by the inclusion of questions on ethnicity at the 1991 and 2001 Censuses. Findings from the 2001 Census for England are shown in Table 3.1, which points to a number of interesting features about the ethnic composition of the English population. First, the overall number of people in minority groups is relatively low compared with countries such as the USA (only 13 per cent in total, and 9 per cent if just non-white groups are considered). Second, the considerable diversity in the ethnic backgrounds of those in the minority groups is underestimated by the broad categories shown. Third, an examination of the ethnic categories reveals close connections between New Commonwealth countries and ethnic minority groups in the UK. Not shown in the table (the data were not available at the time of writing) is that a significant proportion of the non-white ethnic minority UK population are migrants (around half at the time of the 1991 Census), though this varies across specific groups reflecting both period of migration (see later) and patterns of fertility.

The last two points indicate that in order to understand ethnicity in the UK we need to analyse the patterns of inward migration. Briefly, one can characterise the migration pattern of non-white minority groups as a phenomenon of the post-World War II period. In the period prior to and surrounding World War II, most immigration into the UK was of white populations. For some time there has been

35

Table 3.1 Ethnic composition of English population

Ethnic group	Number/1000	Per cent
White British	45534	87.0
White Irish	642	1.3
Other White	1345	2.7
Black Caribbean (incl. mixed)	801	1.6
Black African (incl. mixed)	559	1.1
Other Black	96	0.2
Indian Asian	1037	2.1
Pakistani Asian	715	1.4
Bangladeshi Asian	281	0.6
Other Asian	241	0.5
Mixed White and Asian	189	0.4
Chinese	227	0.5
Other (incl. other mixed)	375	0.7

Source: 2001 Census

significant migration from Ireland and in the first half of the twentieth century migrants to the UK included those fleeing persecution in Nazi Germany and the Soviet Union. Although small numbers of non-white people lived in the UK prior to World War II (mainly in London and the ports on the west coast of the UK – Bristol, Cardiff, Liverpool, Glasgow – and primarily related to the slave trade), most of the non-white migration was driven by the post-war economic boom and consequent need for labour, a need that could be filled from Commonwealth countries – primarily countries in the Caribbean and Indian subcontinent.

This immigration from New Commonwealth countries lasted from the passage of the British Nationality Act in 1948, reaching a peak in the late 1950s and early 1960s, and then decreased following the Immigration Acts of 1962, 1968 and 1971; the former curtailing immigration from the Caribbean and the latter Acts curtailing immigration from the Indian subcontinent (Owen 2003). This 'economic' migration was followed by migration of spouses and children and sometimes older relatives in a climate when the legislation regulating entry into the UK became increasingly restrictive. Migration from these countries was not evenly spread over time. Immigration from the Caribbean and India occurred throughout the 1950s and 1960s, peaking in the early 1960s; that from Pakistan largely occurred in the 1970s; immigration from Bangladesh occurred mainly in the late 1970s and early 1980s; while that from Hong Kong occurred in the 1980s and 1990s. In addition there was a notable flow of immigrants from East Africa in the late 1960s and early 1970s, made up of migrants from India to East Africa who were subsequently expelled. Over the past 15 years, migration to the UK has taken a very different form, largely being made up of refugees, predominantly from African countries, the Middle East, countries such as Sri Lanka, and more recently those from eastern Europe and the former Yugoslavia.

The pattern of migration described above means the vast majority of older non-white ethnic minority people in the UK are first generation migrants. A crucial issue is, then, how the migration experience, most particularly the economic and social climate into which ethnic minority people arrived, shaped their lives as they grew older. How has it affected economic fortunes, health and, perhaps most importantly, a sense of citizenship, belonging and the formation of communities? The fact that the majority of non-white migration occurred in the post-war period also means that ethnic minority populations in the UK have a young age profile. Data from the 2001 Census show that those below compulsory school-leaving age form about a fifth of the white British population, compared with almost a third of the non-white ethnic minority population. In contrast, while around 17 per cent of the white British population were aged 65 or older at the 2001 Census, this was only around 6 per cent for the non-white ethnic minority groups. Differences in age profiles also varied across ethnic minority groups, with, for example, the Pakistani and Bangladeshi populations having a younger profile than the Indian population and the Black Caribbean population having the oldest profile (even if the Black Other group – who are likely to be second generation Black Caribbean people – are included).

So, the young adults who migrated in the 1950s, 1960s and 1970s are only now reaching older ages. As such, their experiences of ageing are and will be unique. They are a non-white migrant generation that made a major contribution to the rebuilding of the post-World War II UK economy, but also faced economic and social exclusion. They had a range of experiences that migrants before them did not face and that will be markedly different for their children.

Given the relative youth of ethnic minority populations in the UK, it is perhaps not surprising that there has not been extensive research on the circumstances of older ethnic minority people. There has, of course, been considerable research on the social, economic and health experiences of ethnic minority people generally, which has mapped the extent of inequality faced by ethnic minority people and how this may well vary across groups, generations and gender (Modood et al. 1997; Nazroo 2001; Mason 2003). The research undertaken on older ethnic minority people has largely focused on health and social care (Cooper et al. 2000; Lowdell et al. 2000). Here the suggestion has been that older ethnic minority people face multiple hazard (Blakemore and Boneham 1993; Ebrahim 1996), or double or triple jeopardy (Mays 1983; Norman 1985) as a consequence of both their ethnic minority status and their older age.

Rather than simply mapping dimensions of inequality across ethnic groups, the study reported here used the concept of 'quality of life' to understand the impact of the circumstances of older ethnic minority people on their well-being. Many researchers have noted the lack of a theoretical base to the concept of quality of life (Hornquist 1982; Gill and Feinstein 1994; Bowling 1997; Hunt, 1997; Smith 2000). In its absence a common approach has been to see quality of life as the assemblage of a number of dimensions that are likely to be relevant to it, such as health, finances, neighbourhood and social networks. In this study we adopt a different approach that builds on the work of Higgs et al. (2003) and Hyde et al. (2003), and which treats quality of life as a phenomenon distinct from its potential influences. That is, we treat health, finances, neighbourhood, social networks and so forth as potential influences on quality of life, rather than as component factors. In part we adopted this approach because it is likely that the nature and relevance of particular influences on quality of life will be culturally informed and, consequently, vary across ethnic groups.

The study

The study used both secondary analysis of quantitative data and the collection and analysis of qualitative data. The quantitative data were drawn from both the 1999 Health Survey for England (HSE) (Erens et al. 2001; Nazroo 2004) and the Fourth National Survey of Ethnic Minorities (FNS) (Modood et al. 1997; Bajekal et al. 2003), both large representative surveys of ethnic minority and white people. The data contained in these studies tapped a range of characteristics, including demographic, economic, social and health. The data were used in this study to provide a description of the circumstances – the influences on quality of life – of older ethnic minority people and to draw comparisons between them and the majority population.

The highly subjective nature of quality of life and its great potential variability in meaning across different ethnic groups made it crucial for us to include qualitative research alongside the analysis of the quantitative data. For this part of the study we drew a purposive subsample from the FNS (see Grewal et al. 2004). In selecting people to include in the qualitative work, our expectation was that using ethnic minority groups that are as homogeneous as possible would maximise the possibility of finding differences between them. Also, we considered the inclusion of a white English group to be crucial, both to provide a point of comparison (ensuring that difference is not essentialised to supposed racial or ethnic characteristics) and so that English ethnicity itself could be a focus of investigation. The sampling also covered dimensions of age, gender and class. A total of 73 in-depth qualitative interviews were carried out with respondents aged between 60 and 74 years from four ethnic groups (Jamaican Caribbean, Gujarati Indian Hindu, Punjabi Pakistani and white English).

Data were collected through semi-structured in-depth interviews, which began by collecting family, education, residential, employment, and health histories. They then moved on to current circumstances and concluded by discussing attitudes to ageing. The interviews were conducted in the language(s) of the respondent's choice, imperative in enabling full expression of complicated ideas and emotion (Elam et al. 1999; Nazroo and Grewal 2002).

Ethnicity, inequality and age: a description

Here we will describe the circumstances of older ethnic minority people in the UK, covering health, economic position, geographical environment and social networks.

Health

The health data shown here are drawn from the 1999 HSE, so include a white minority group and cover ages from two years upwards. The 1999 HSE covered a large range of both general and disease-specific indicators of respondents' health. Here only one of these indicators is considered, a question asking respondents to rate their current general health (or their child's current general health if she or he is aged less than 12) on a five-point scale: very good, good, fair, bad and very bad. (The pattern for other health indicators included in the HSE show a similar overall pattern.) In Figure 3.1 the scale has been dichotomised into good versus fair or bad and the proportion of respondents reporting fair or bad health by ethnicity and age is shown. The figure is striking; ethnic inequalities in health increase markedly with age. The small differences in early childhood disappear in late childhood and early adulthood, but then reappear in early middle age and grow throughout the rest of adulthood, meaning that differences are very marked for the early old age cohort. The profiles of the Caribbean and Indian groups are similar to each other, and show a worsening in health in comparison with the white English group from the mid-thirties to the mid-forties cohort onwards, while the Pakistani and Bangladeshi groups have a markedly worse profile than other groups, with differences emerging from the mid-twenties cohort onwards. The group with the poorest reported health throughout, Bangladeshi people, have rates around 50 per cent higher than those for white English people from the mid-forties cohort onwards. It is worth noting that the white minority group has a very similar profile to the white English group throughout the age span, and that for the Chinese group is close to these two.

Economic position

The data on economic position (economic activity, occupational class and household income) shown here are also drawn from the 1999 HSE.

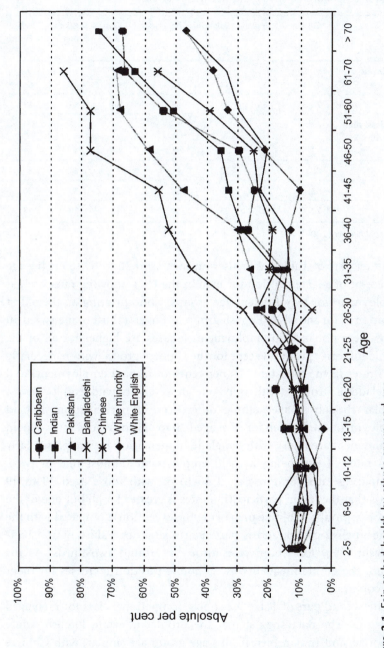

Figure 3.1 Fair or bad health by ethnic group and age
Source: Nazroo (2004)

Table 3.2 Economic activity and occupational class

	Caribbean	Indian	Pakistani	Bangladeshi	Chinese	White minority	White English
	%	%	%	%	%	%	%
Employed							
Men aged 50–65	42	57	31	16	62	47	63
Men aged 30–49	74	86	78	55	88	84	88
RG class, men aged 50–65							
I/II	12	37	26	9	49	43	39
IIInm	8	9	12	4	1	6	8
IIIm	53	27	29	39	35	30	36
IV/V	27	27	33	48	15	20	17

Source: Nazroo (2004)

The first part of Table 3.2 focuses on men aged 30 to 65 (65 is the age of receipt of a state pension for men in the UK), showing rates of paid employment for two different age groups. Concentrating on the oldest group first, for the white English group just over a third of men aged 50 to 65 were not in paid employment. Figures are higher for all of the ethnic minority groups, except for the Chinese group, with particularly high rates in the Pakistani (70 per cent not in paid employment) and Bangladeshi groups (with only one in seven in paid employment). Similar though smaller ethnic differences in participation in paid employment can be seen for men aged 30 to 49 (for whom rates of paid employment are high), with Bangladeshi men again having particularly high rates of not being in paid employment (almost one in two). Comparing rates for those aged 50 to 65 with those aged 30 to 49 shows that the fall in participation rates is greater for all but one of the minority groups (Chinese men being the exception) compared with the white English group, and is particularly large for Pakistani and Bangladeshi men, for whom rates drop by around two-thirds. As for health, the ethnic inequality in economic position increases for older age cohorts.

The second part of Table 3.2 shows occupational class for men aged 50 to 65. The data suggest that the profiles of white English, white minority, and Indian men in this age group are similar, with Chinese men better off and Caribbean, Pakistani and particularly Bangladeshi men worse off. The striking difference between women (not shown in the table) is the level of participation in paid employment. Analysis of the 1999 HSE show that among women of working age around a quarter of Caribbean, white minority and white English women are economically inactive, compared with just over a third of Indian and Chinese women and around four-fifths of Pakistani and Bangladeshi women. These figures increase for all groups if women aged 50 to 60 are considered (60 is currently the age of receipt of a state pension for women in the UK), but the broad pattern remains the same. The most stark finding is that only 2 per cent of Bangladeshi women in the 50 to 60 age group are in paid employment compared with around 10 per cent of Pakistani women, just over a third of Indian women and close to two-thirds of Caribbean, white minority and white English women (Nazroo 2004).

Figure 3.2 shows household income from all sources for households with one or more members aged 50 or older split into tertiles on the basis of the general population distribution (of all ages) and equivalised to account for variations in household size using the McClemens scoring system (Erens et al. 2001). The figure shows that the two white groups are equivalent, with the Indian as well as the Caribbean group being worse off, and the Pakistani as well as the Bangladeshi group particularly poorly off. Three-quarters of the Pakistani group and more than 90 per cent of the Bangladeshi group were in the bottom income tertile. In terms of the top income tertile, the Chinese group is equivalent to the two white groups, but it also has substantially more households in this age group in the bottom tertile.

Quality of neighbourhood

Principal components factor analysis (Kim and Mueller 1979; Bajekal et al. 2004) of questions in the FNS was used to provide a rating of perceptions of the local area for respondents aged 45 to 74 in four ethnic groups, Caribbean, Indian, Pakistani and white. The factor analysis identified ratings for two dimensions of the local area: amenities (for example, shops, schools, public transport, leisure facilities, places of work, ease of getting to work) and crime/environment (for example, vandalism, car thefts, burglaries, assaults, safety, rubbish, nuisance children, graffiti, unkempt areas, dog mess, traffic and parking).

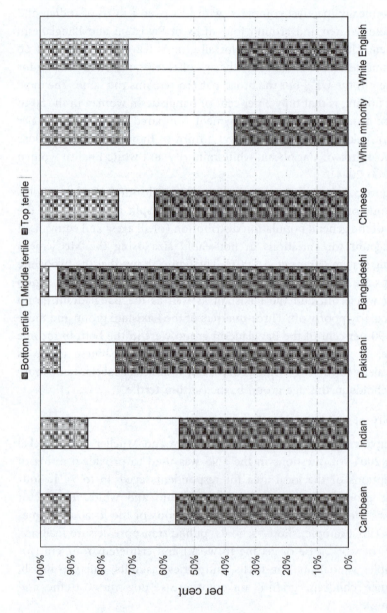

Figure 3.2 Equivalised household income: households with one or more person aged 50 or older
Source: Nazroo (2004)

Table 3.3 Percentage of the population with a score equal to or better than the white median for reported local crime and environment

		Caribbean	Indian	Pakistani
Total		53	64	45
Men	Age 45–54	60	67	52
	Age 55–64	38	58	27
	Age 65–74	57	62	41
Women	Age 45–54	43	62	51
	Age 55–64	65	71	47
	Age 65–74	35	54	[41]

Percentages based on less than 30 counts in brackets [].
Source: Bajekal et al. (2004)

The overall ratings of crime and the quality of the physical environment were significantly poorer for the Pakistani group compared with the white group, and significantly better for the Indian group. Table 3.3 gives a sense of the size of this difference by showing the population proportions with a score equal to or better than the white group median score. The total row in the table shows that 64 per cent of people of Indian origin had a score equal to or higher than the median (50 per cent) score for the white group, compared with 45 per cent of the Pakistani group. For the Caribbean group 53 per cent of respondents had a score equal to or better than the white group median score, a non-significant difference. With advancing age, Pakistani men and women continued to be more likely to report problems with crime and the quality of the physical environment relative to the white people of the same age and gender.

In contrast, the overall rating for the availability of local amenities was significantly better for all three ethnic minority groups relative to the white group. The total row in Table 3.4 confirms that proportionately more ethnic minority people had scores higher than the median score for the white population. For instance, 81 per cent of people of Pakistani origin had a score equal to or higher than the median (50 per cent) score for the white group. Overall, the population proportions above the white median cut-point were highest for Pakistani people, and successively lower for the Caribbean and Indian groups. The other columns in the table show that this overall rank position by ethnicity

Table 3.4 Percentage of the population with a score equal to or better than the white median for reported quality of local amenities

		Caribbean	Indian	Pakistani
Total		72	69	81
Men	Age 45–54	73	68	75
	Age 55–64	70	80	72
	Age 65–74	84	69	88
Women	Age 45–54	68	60	78
	Age 55–64	79	77	91
	Age 65–74	67	60	[86]

Percentages based on less than 30 counts in brackets [].
Source: Bajekal et al. (2004)

was consistently observed across successive age bands and for men and women, indicating that the perception of availability of amenities locally did not alter with advancing age or by gender for any of the four groups.

In addition to these self-reports of the local neighbourhood, we examined national, objective, estimates of relative deprivation for the same areas, as measured by the Index of Deprivation 2000 (ID2000) overall score and the ID2000 score for access to services (shops, GP, school, etc.). The ID2000 does not have a separate domain relating to crime or physical environment (DETR 2000). Table 3.5 shows that the perception of the local neighbourhood as reported by the FNS respondents is in sharp contrast to and indeed inversely related to 'formal' estimates of relative deprivation for the same areas in terms of both the ID2000 overall score and the service access score. At one end

Table 3.5 ID2000 amenities and overall score for areas rated by FNS respondents

	White	Caribbean	Indian	Pakistani
Means (lower is better)				
ID2000 access to amenities (*−1)	0.63	0.97	0.74	0.97
ID2000 overall score	21.8	39.7	30.8	50.1

Source: Bajekal et al. (2004)

of the spectrum, Pakistani residents living in wards classified as the most deprived and with the poorest access to services rated their neighbourhoods highly on the amenities factor. At the other end of the spectrum, the white group living in relatively more affluent areas perceived the quality of local amenities in their neighbourhoods to be a lot worse than any of the ethnic minority groups.

Social networks and participation

Factor analysis of questions in the FNS was also used to provide a rating of frequency of contact with family networks and community participation for respondents aged 45 to 74 in the same four ethnic groups: Caribbean, Indian, Pakistani and white. The family network factor covered questions on frequency of seeing relatives, writing to relatives and speaking on the phone to relatives, while that for community participation covered membership of organisations, voluntary activities, providing informal care and membership of political parties and trade unions.

Contact with family was significantly higher in Indian and Pakistani groups compared with the white group. Table 3.6 shows the percentage of people scoring the same as or higher than the median (50 per cent) score for the white sample. The Pakistani group ranked first (79 per cent), followed by the Indian (73 per cent), Caribbean (67 per cent) and the white (50 per cent) groups. The same pattern was observed for

Table 3.6 Percentage of the population with a score equal to or more frequent than the white median for reported contact with family networks

		Caribbean	Indian	Pakistani
Total		67	73	79
Men	Age 45–54	74	78	77
	Age 55–64	63	78	81
	Age 65–74	54	69	83
Women	Age 45–54	24	23	18
	Age 55–64	70	61	75
	Age 65–74	68	75	[75]

Percentages based on less than 30 counts in brackets [].
Source: Bajekal et al. (2004)

men across all age groups, and for women aged 55 and over. In contrast, women in the youngest age band (45–54) in all three ethnic minority groups have markedly lower levels of familial contact relative to women in the white group. These differences do not reach statistical significance because of small numbers. It is worth noting that in general in all four ethnic groups contact with family declined significantly with the passing of each decade from age 45.

Overall levels of community participation were significantly higher for the white group, but did not vary much between the ethnic minority groups. For all groups, the distribution was highly skewed, with most informants to the survey reporting no active participation on either the formal (political parties, trades union) or informal (voluntary work, informal care) types of community engagement. As a result, and as shown in Table 3.7, the percentage distributions above the white group's median score are very similar across ethnic minority groups. There was considerably greater variation by age and gender. Overall, participation among women was significantly lower than for men. After state retirement age (65–74), Caribbean women and Pakistani men have higher numbers participating in community activities than other groups. Pre-retirement, men in all the ethnic minority groups have markedly lower levels of social participation than white men. The same holds true for women aged 45 to 54, but increases to levels similar to those of women in the white group for the 55 to 64 age group.

Table 3.7 Percentage of the population with a score equal to or higher than the white median for reported community participation

		Caribbean	Indian	Pakistani
Total		54	55	53
Men	Age 45–54	19	16	9
	Age 55–64	11	7	1
	Age 65–74	45	51	65
Women	Age 45–54	15	5	1
	Age 55–64	53	54	48
	Age 65–74	77	53	[56]

Percentages based on less than 30 counts in brackets [].
Source: Bajekal et al. (2004)

Summary

This description of the position of older ethnic minority people in comparison with their white peers is more complex than suggested by claims of multiple hazard or double/triple jeopardy. External measures of economic position (economic activity, occupational class and household income) and local area deprivation scores (ID2000), along with a subjective assessment of health, suggest significant disadvantage for ethnic minority people, and a disadvantage that increases with age. If a hierarchy of disadvantage is drawn, Bangladeshi and Pakistani people are the worst off, followed respectively by Caribbean, Indian and white people. However, other perhaps more subjective assessments of circumstances are less clear. Respondents' ratings of the quality of the local area in terms of crime and physical activity, and scores for community participation, do not show a clear advantage for white people. Respondents' ratings of local amenities show a clear advantage for ethnic minority people, as do those for participation in family networks. The contrasting pattern of the ID2000 amenities score and the respondents' ratings of their local amenities highlights the possibility that external assessments may miss key dimensions of people's lives and, in the case of ethnic minority people, dimensions that bring positive elements to the quality of their lives. The next section of this chapter uses the qualitative part of our study to explore this further by showing how one of the contributors to quality of life identified by respondents, having a role, depends on both external factors and the agency of people within migrant communities.

A deeper understanding of ethnic inequalities – the case of roles, gender and quality of life

A central feature of the qualitative side of this study was to explore the factors that respondents felt brought quality to their lives. Interestingly there was great consistency in the factors that were identified by respondents in all four of the ethnic groups, although the way these factors featured in people's lives varied by ethnicity (Grewal et al. 2004). The factors discussed by respondents can be structured under the following broad themes: having a role; support networks; income and wealth; health; having time; and independence. Here we focus on having a role – something on which immense importance was placed by respondents from all four ethnic groups included in this part of the study and its relationship to other dimensions, in order to illustrate the importance of understanding both the subjective and objective dimensions of people's lives when considering quality of life, and how this relates to both ethnicity and migration. Within the broad category of having a role, we more specifically focus on paid work, role in the community, and role as a parent and grandparent.

Role through paid work

The role as a paid worker was experienced in a number of ways. Among those still in paid work, some reported not being able to afford to retire if they wanted to maintain their existing standard of living, or felt that they had to continue working in order to improve their pension package. For these respondents the paid work role did not bring quality to their lives. In contrast, others enjoyed their work – it brought them some fulfilment – so did not wish to retire, or after retirement they took up the opportunity to return to their former profession in some form of part-time consultancy capacity. These contrasting positions related to class and thereby to ethnicity. The option to return to work in a consultancy capacity after retirement was an experience concentrated among white professional men. For some, especially those who had retired from manual work, retirement brought a sense of being 'delighted for the rest' from arduous labour. For example, Punjabi Pakistani men did not, on the whole, describe paid work enthusiastically. Perhaps not surprisingly given the quantitative findings described above, for these respondents retirement commonly appeared to have been forced on them by ill health or long-term unemployment. In this context, those Punjabi Pakistani men who did express regret about not having paid work did so mostly in relation to its financial implications.

For those ethnic minority respondents who did describe having enjoyed their work, this was more in the context of having something to do, rather than anything about the inherent quality of the job. Even where long-term ill health had preceded retirement, the end of paid work led some in all of the ethnic groups to have feelings of loss of identity and purpose. Such a sentiment was expressed by a Punjabi Pakistani man who, despite having been out of work for almost ten years due to ill health, nevertheless felt a sense of loss on retirement: 'When a man retires he is finished, what else is left of life?' The loss of self-esteem was reported with particular bitterness by those who had faced 'forced' retirement and had subsequently not been able to find other paid work. This view, common among white English men, is illustrated in the quote below:

> Really when you're my age you can't get jobs easily so I've been forced to retire ... I'm not happy about it, I don't like it ... I searched a long time ... And it's very frustrating because ... I think it's wrong-headed ... [at] 55 (a) you've got tremendous experience, (b) you're level headed and (c) we're not threatening anybody in their jobs ... we're not quite that eager to get ahead so we've got a lot to offer

So, what is clear is that both the opportunity to work in the years before and after the state pension age, and the satisfaction obtained from work, were structured by the location of people in the labour force. This related to class, gender and ethnicity – with those in more professional jobs getting greater reward from their work, having more opportunity to work up to and past state retirement age, and being less likely to be forced out of work because of ill health.

Role through community

Undertaking voluntary work was a popular role and one that was often acquired through the 'community'. However, this meant different things for ethnic minority and white English older people. For white English older people this usually involved doing voluntary work for a national or a local charity with a specific issue focus, for example, old age, disability, or housing. For ethnic minority people voluntary work tended to be based in the local ethnic community, and was typically channelled through religion. A possible explanation for this difference in the nature of the voluntary work can be found in the settlement patterns of ethnic minority older people and how this shaped their relationships with the local community. Settlement patterns following migration meant that ethnic minority people tended to set up home in areas where other migrants lived, or they moved to such an area because of the local facilities such as places of worship. Further, there was evidence that members of these 'reconstituted' communities also found employment together in local industries. Hence, for ethnic minority people the work community and the local community were typically either the same, or there were overlaps between them. Both were involved in the composition of the community, and there were opportunities for voluntary work that focused on the local ethnic minority community generally rather than a specific issue in the community.

In contrast, white English older people often worked in an area some distance from where they lived and the distance increased if they moved, for example, to be nearer grandchildren, or to a smaller house following retirement. Therefore, the work community and the local community were typically two separate entities.

For ethnic minority older people, voluntary work was often channelled through religion and there was evidence of gender demarcations in roles here. For Punjabi Pakistani respondents following the Islamic faith, this often gave men an active role in the community, for example, teaching in mosques, taking part in organised religious debates, advising others, and opening doors at the mosque five times a day for the *namaz* [formal prayer]. For Muslim women religion also provided a function; often their day was structured around reading the *namaz* five times a day (as was that of the men). This tended to be carried out inside the house and that, consequently, did not necessarily have an element of community interaction attached.

Some Jamaican respondents also spoke of taking on an educational role by running prayer classes, advising others in the community and visiting those unable to attend the church due to ill health in their homes, or at hospital. In line with the Islamic faith, following Christianity lent structure to Jamaican people's lives by, for example, requiring them to attend services at a church and to prepare for prayer meetings. However, unlike Punjabi Pakistani respondents, there did not appear to be a gender difference in the take-up of such activities. The Gujarati experience also provided a structure to the day, for example, bathing, lighting a lamp and praying, but unlike the other two there was little evidence of this being used as a route to active roles in the community; nor was there any indication of a gender demarcation in this.

As a result of the local nature of their voluntary work, it followed that respondents from the ethnic minority sample usually participated in charitable work to assist with the social, educational, emotional and practical needs of their own ethnic community. The types of voluntary work undertaken across ethnic groups included: an advisor in a domestic violence support group; a school governor; a fund raiser for the Gujarat earthquake disaster appeal; a community liaison officer working with the police. These roles offered the individuals an opportunity to give something back, to feel useful and valuable. In other words it was a way of continuing to make a contribution at older ages.

Role as parent and grandparent

Relationships with children and grandchildren provided a range of roles that again showed some variation by ethnicity and gender, and that related to roles in the community. In cases where older people lived with their son or daughter, and sometimes their son's or daughter's children as well, they often took on a parenting role that mirrored the one they had played when their own children were younger, such as the mother cooking and cleaning and the father chauffeuring. Within the multigenerational households there was evidence of gender affecting the types of roles that were played. Men tended to take on the role as the head of the household, with a Punjabi Pakistani man describing himself as the 'decision maker', and another as the one who has 'control of all the [household] money', while the women adopted, or continued to play, the caring role. There were a number of reasons that had led older people to share a house with their offspring. Among them were not being able to afford to live on their own, not wanting to live alone following the death of their partner, or needing to be looked after due to failing health. The latter reason influenced the type of role that they were able to play in the household.

Even where older people did not live with their children, they still had a sense of being responsible for them so that, for example, they wished their children to settle down (and have children) and gave advice and financial and practical support to them. Some Punjabi Pakistani respondents described the sense that they were responsible for their children, even after the children were married and had their own families, as an 'obligation'. They felt an obligation to ensure that their children lived their lives in a certain way. This was linked to their religious faith and the fact that as longstanding members of a local ethnically defined community their children's behaviour could have an effect on their own standing in the community.

In relation to grandchildren, three types of roles emerged. None was exclusive to a particular ethnic group. First was the childminding role, which varied from full-time parenting in the grandchild's early years to part-time parenting during holidays. Second was the 'having fun with' role that included, for example, day trips, playing football in the park, going to the cinema, and so on. Third was an educational teacher role. For ethnic minority respondents, the latter role involved teaching and maintaining 'the old ways'. The type of grandparenting role adopted was often influenced by locality, which itself was strongly related to ethnicity. For example, those living with their grandchildren in multigenerational households tended to be the Gujarati and Punjabi Pakistani respondents. Cohabitation meant that there was a higher degree of day-to-day involvement in their grandchildren's lives, though not necessarily in bringing them up. For example, in some multigenerational households looking after the children remained the responsibility of the parents. Grandparents were responsible for educating their grandchildren about religion and preserving their culture. This preservation of culture was seen as an important role by many ethnic minority respondents, and one that mapped onto their roles as elders within a local ethnically defined community.

Bringing the dimensions together

The value to respondents of having a fulfilling role was clear. But the types of roles available within the domains described, and more importantly that the older person is able to take up, are fundamentally shaped by ethnicity, in part through the relationships between ethnicity health, occupation and income. As numerous studies have revealed, and as our earlier descriptive data showed, older people from ethnic minority groups fare poorly in these domains (Blakemore and Boneham 1993; Smaje 1995; Nazroo 2001, 2004; Bajekal et al. 2004).

In terms of health, a decline in the ability to function, both cognitively and physically, is associated with a decline in other activities and consequently influences the types of social roles an individual can play. A core theme in the accounts of the respondents to this study was the significance of a decline in health to their ability to perform the roles and activities that they wanted to do, or were obliged to do. Poor health had an impact on the ability to engage in paid work, to engage in community activities such as voluntary work, to maintain friendships and to fulfil roles within the household and families, such as running a home or grandparenting.

An important determinant of living standards in old age is employment status prior to retirement, because inequalities experienced in the labour market are reflected in economic inequalities in retirement (Walker 1981). We have shown in our quantitative findings that ethnic minority older people are at much greater risk of poverty than white English older people (Bajekal et al. 2004; Nazroo 2004), perhaps because the former are generally more likely to have had lower earnings or experienced long-term unemployment during their working lives (Fru and Glendenning 1988; Modood et al. 1997). Those in low-paid work are far less likely to contribute towards a private pension and the length of employment and type of occupation also affect the value of any occupational pension received. Older women from ethnic minority groups can be further disadvantaged. They are even more likely to be in low-paid work or to not have had jobs at all. Not surprisingly, in the accounts of respondents in this study there were also clear descriptions of a good economic position allowing respondents to enjoy their old age, free from financial concerns and able to participate in the activities that brought them enjoyment and rewards (Grewal et al. 2004). These were more typical of older white people.

For ethnic minority people, limited financial resources and poor health had an impact on the role as a 'wise elder', to whom family, friends and wider community came for advice, because for some this role came literally at a price. For example, Punjabi Pakistani and Gujarati respondents explained that as heads of households, or as respected elders in the community, their status brought with it financial expectations, such as giving money at weddings, helping others financially with costs for funerals in India or Pakistan and making religious donations. The quote below illustrates the dilemmas that they face when they struggled to meet these expectations:

> I know so many people in [name of city] and there is no week without
> having to attend two or three weddings because they call me and if you
> don't go then there is no respect and they think he didn't come because
> of the money but they don't know your financial position, the govern-
> ment doesn't give you money for the weddings.

The type of job respondents had also had implications beyond financial resources. Keeping a role by continuing in employment in some form up to and beyond state retirement age was an option that seemed to be more likely for white English than ethnic minority people, perhaps because the former were more likely to be in professional occupations. For the latter, employment tended to be concentrated in manual jobs that, due to their physicality, have no scope for continuing into old age, or to a return post-retirement, for example, in a consultant capacity. Notwithstanding the opportunity that some took up to continue in some capacity in the family business, for example, working in a shop, for ethnic minority people a 'work-type' role was more likely to come through their relationship with an ethnically specific community.

There appeared to be an influence of migration on the types or ways that roles developed through the community. For white English people a voluntary 'work-type' role usually means participating in charity-based voluntary work at both a national and local level. For ethnic minority people, voluntary work is more likely to be channelled through their local ethnic community or religion, often being conducted via church, temple, mosque or community centre. Another push for a significant role of religion in the lives of ethnic minority people can also be found in their migration history. Ethnic minority respondents recalled the lack of appropriate places of worship on their arrival. Consequently, they had been part of the process of establishing such a resource. Thus their involvement and connection with religion was organic, often with a great deal of personal investment. With retirement, or children leaving home, and the resulting free time, there was a need for alternative roles and religion offered one option.

For Gujarati and Punjabi Pakistani respondents there was an additional purpose to religion. There was a perception that second generation members of their communities were becoming assimilated into the British way of life. Changes such as increased social mobility among second generation people, which sometimes resulted in a geographical scattering of families, strengthened this perception. So older people used their faith as a means to maintain and pass on cultural values and ethnic identity to future generations. This could be interpreted as a Third Age activity, where Laslett (1989: 193) refers to 'the preservation of prosperity of our cultural inheritance, material as well as intellectual and literacy'. Jamaican people did not report this in the same way, which suggests that the preservation of language, and perhaps religion, may be a motivating factor.

As suggested by the discussion of ethnic differences in economic resources, differences in life histories, structured by the experience of migration, play a central role in explaining ethnic differences in the resources to acquire roles. For example, one of the roles that the family can offer is as a grandparent and it is a role that may bring a lot of joy and pleasure. For Pakistani, Jamaican and Gujarati respondents, experience of migration, migration patterns and settlement patterns can determine the type of, if any, grandparenting role that they can expect. A consequence of migration is that families are split and (re)constructed once in England. There is evidence among Jamaican respondents of children remaining in Jamaica or migrating to another country. The result of this is that the 'special' relationship with grandchildren cannot be developed when financial constraints do not allow frequent contact. Gujarati and Punjabi Pakistani people had a different experience, with nuclear families not split by migration. Further there is evidence of multigenerational households in these groups, which means that grandparents can be living with their grandchildren and therefore have much more time with them. In contrast, the absence of disruption to families as a consequence of international migration means that the grandparenting experience of white English older people is more predictable and one that typically took the form of 'leisure grandparenting'; for example, having a fixed amount of time to take them to the cinema or to undertake an activity. But for some the frequency of this was disrupted by migration within the UK, with sometimes quite large distances between respondents and their children and grandchildren.

Conclusion

There are marked ethnic inequalities in the areas of economic position and health, inequalities that have been documented elsewhere, although they may be changing, in form at least, across generations (Modood et al. 1997; Mason 2003). The evidence we have reported here suggests that ethnic inequalities in health and economic position are at their greatest for older people. The extent of the economic disadvantage faced by some ethnic minority groups at older ages is extreme. For example, fewer than one in six Bangladeshi and one in three Pakistani men aged 50 to 65 is in paid employment, compared with almost two-thirds of white English men aged 50 to 65. More than 90 per cent of Bangladeshi and three-quarters of Pakistani households with one or more members aged 50 or more are in the bottom income tertile, compared with only just over a third of equivalent white English households. Similarly, ethnic inequalities in health at older ages are very large: for those aged between 50 and 70 less than one-fifth of Bangladeshi and less than a third of Pakistani people describe their health as better than fair, compared with around two-thirds of white English people. The significance of this cannot be overestimated. Both ethnic minority and white respondents described how their activities and, consequently, quality of life were severely circumscribed by health and financial problems. Here it is important to recognise that older ethnic minority people do not uniquely face these inequalities and that they are not uniformly experienced in ethnic minority populations, but they are far more common.

The origins of the economic disadvantage of older ethnic minority people undoubtedly lay in their post-migration experiences, with employment opportunities on the whole restricted to jobs with poorer pay, poorer security and often with more limited pension rights (Brodie 1996). Even those who were recruited into professional occupations such as medicine faced considerable disadvantage in employment (Kyriakides and Virdee 2003). It is also worth recognising that the impact of the decline of manufacturing industries in the UK in the 1980s was particularly significant for this generation of ethnic minority people, many of whom spent the period before their pension age unemployed, or unable to work because of poor health. There is considerable evidence suggesting that ethnic inequalities in health are driven by economic inequalities (Nazroo 2001); evidence that shows how closely related experiences of poverty, unemployment and poor health are and evidence that, it is suggested, shows the significance of racism and discrimination to the life chances of those ethnic minority people who migrated to the UK in the 1950s and 1960s (Nazroo 2003).

This portrayal of disadvantage does not, however, fully capture the experiences of older ethnic minority people. As we have shown, across other dimensions of their lives ethnic minority older people fare as well as or better than their white counterparts. Most notably, ethnic minority older people appear to do relatively well in terms of community, social and family networks, both in terms of their global quantitative assessments and in terms of their descriptions of the role opportunities and status that such networks offer them. Again this can perhaps best be understood in relation to the experiences of a migrant generation. Respondents described the (re)building of ethnic communities post-migration, a rebuilding that was aided by close settlement patterns and employment in local industries. The investment of this migrant generation in the building of a local ethnic community is something that many seemed able to draw on in their older ages – even if for some it also carried obligations. Of course the development of such communities occurred in the face of considerable local and national hostility (Kyriakides and Virdee 2003). It is here that the need becomes apparent to consider the situation of ethnic minority older people not just in terms of the ways their lives have been structured by economic and social forces, but also in terms of how this structuring has been resisted by individuals and groups. The building, in response to post-migration hostility and exclusion, of communities that protect individuals and offer roles in the context of ongoing significant economic hardship and poor health has evidently done much to enhance the lives of at least some ethnic minority older people.

4

Environment, identity and old age – quality of life or a life of quality?

Leonie Kellaher, Sheila M. Peace and Caroline Holland

Introduction

The study of environment and identity in old age reported here (Peace et al. 2003) started with two implicit assumptions: first, that the material and social environment grounds everyday living; second, that these day-to-day experiences can support or compromise identity, which it is acknowledged (Gardner 2002; Hockey and James 2003) is mutable rather than stable. The missing link is the nature of the dynamic that connects environment to identity and quality. Our previous research in the special setting of residential care homes showed that restricted environmental experience could compromise the sense of self, and that this in turn is associated with reduced quality of life for older residents (Willcocks et al. 1987). Consequently, the research undertaken for this new study has aimed to explore the dynamic involved for older people who live in a wider range of living environments and neighbourhoods than our earlier research. The present settings of our informants covered the very special residential and care home environment, through sheltered and special housing, and the wide variety of ordinary domestic settings of the majority of older people in UK. Thus, our data reflect 'historical' accounts of different environments as well as a cross-sectional view of responses in old age to the possibilities and limitations of different settings revealed in the changing contexts of ageing.

The title of the project, 'Environment and Identity in Later Life:

a cross-setting study', hints at the inner and external worlds that are implied in daily life. The interaction of these worlds has been our primary concern. The fixed items and domains which underpinned earlier quality of life studies become secondary to the more dynamic mechanism or sets of strategies that older individuals bring into play as they keep themselves going and, though few actually used such terms, make a *life of quality*. Trajectories or pathways linking the inner and external worlds that make environment begin to come into focus through informants' accounts of their homes, neighbourhoods, lives and hopes. Broadly, these show how people try to manoeuvre themselves into positions that are comfortable both physically and socially and maximise their influence over things both materially and in their networks, however fragile the latter may have become as changes and uncertainty build up with age and over time.

In speaking of internal and external environments we are not making exact alignments with the subjective and objective frames within which quality of life has more traditionally been examined (Willcocks et al. 1987: 122). It could be argued that the ostensibly 'subjective' indicators of quality of life adopted elsewhere (Neugarten et al. 1961; Bradburn 1969; Lawton 1972, 1975) take on an objective complexion when evaluations derived from aggregate scores are imposed on individuals or groups. Such summative analyses sit uncomfortably with the formative evaluations our data suggest are made by older people themselves as they weigh up their lives, their environments and their future life moves. Maintenance of identity and consequent 'quality' appear to rest upon particular and ever-changing appraisals made by older people as they manoeuvre their individual ways through time and place. Their subjective viewpoints, nonetheless, are shaped and tested by constant exposure to the 'objective' realities of the many environments they encounter, which may include material, functional, social and intimate, organisational and legislative environments. The immediate background to this study lies partly in our earlier research on older people in special settings and more recent research on domestic settings (Hanson et al. forthcoming). Equally important, however, have been the analyses of scholars who have made more extensive forays into the questions of person–environment interrelations outlined below. We hope we can add to their work by commenting on issues that have to do with quality.

The policy context

Our study began in the early years of the New Labour administration, following the 'new rightism' of the previous one. Government policy on housing for older people has been set within contexts of ongoing societal and household change and a housing market that had been radically transformed over the previous half century. Some of the social and cultural influences on people and the places where they lived at this time were by no means confined to British society. For example, an ageing society and ageism, privatism in social lives and the privatisation of property and services and gender politics characterised other developed countries. Britain had, however, experienced a sustained period of reduction in the average size of households with large numbers of older people living alone. The expansion of owner occupation coupled with a drastic reduction in the availability of social housing and changes in the provision of residential care places for older people was also particular to the British scene. The development of age-segregated communities, an emphasis on supporting independence in old age and latterly on environmental accessibility and the development of assistive technologies point to other issues involved in providing quality housing for older people (Peace and Holland 2001). At the same time there has been growing attention to older people's rights as citizens and consumers and an interest in involving them in policy development. Against this background the study aimed to introduce into the policy debate some of the implications of the theoretical underpinnings discussed below, and to contribute to the renewed quality debate as it could relate to older people's lives.

The research approach and methodology

The research design for this study reflected the conviction that the complexity of person–environment connection could best be explored through older people speaking about the fine grain of day-to-day environmental experience. It followed that the nature and locus of quality in people's lives was more likely to be uncovered through ethnographic exploration of particular cases than through psychometric or statistical measurement. However, we have considered several measures of quality of life in order to compare the experiential categories that older people might indicate as significant with those generated by established inventories and scales. The development of a new tool for appraising quality of life, validated by older people themselves and relevant across a range of living environments, has arisen out of this juxtaposition of approaches.

For a largely qualitative study, the data is extensive, coming first of all from 9 discussion groups and then from 54 informants who occupied the spectrum of accommodation from ordinary domestic housing to special settings such as sheltered and residential homes. Within each of three location types – metropolitan, urban/suburban, small town/village/semi-rural – different housing styles and tenures were included. A broad interpretation of 'environment' underpinned enquiry with a focus on the dwelling itself, its neighbourhood and wider setting, and the spaces such as gardens that mediate between inside and outside, private and public.

Ethnographic studies with very small numbers of respondents, seen intensively over quite long periods, have already confirmed the complexity of person–environment interaction. Whilst quality of life issues have remained implicit, findings have justified such an intensive methodology. Participant observation, in-depth interviewing, taking housing histories, cognitive mapping, collecting photographic records of domestic and special housing interiors, mapping floor plans and furniture arrangements, taking object inventories and the use of video have been developed as appropriate methods for data collection in this and other studies (Peace 1977; Holland 2001). These approaches have accompanied the recognition that people lay claim to multiple identities (Hockey and James 2003) and they have highlighted both the situational and personal factors that impinge upon the individual. For example, levels of financial resource, weakening of social networks and occasions of age discrimination need to be seen alongside and interwoven with the personal experiences of an ageing individual who may experience increasing levels of morbidity, degrees of social isolation and sensory loss. The cross-tabulation or multiple regression of these 'factors', 'domains' or 'indicators' no longer seems the most useful approach to exploring the deep complexity of everyday life within social and material worlds.

Alongside these methodological issues, the late 1990s also saw the beginnings of greater participation by informants in the research process.

For instance certain groups, particularly younger people with disabilities, experienced the research process as empowering. At the same time policymakers and research funders have insisted on involving service users, sometimes beyond the consultative role and requiring research skills, in the development of services and policies (Peace 2002). Reflecting such developments, our research started with group discussions to identify categories that older people themselves thought were significant for the places where they lived.[1] Topics generated included: defining 'my/our place'; security; routines; comfort and convenience; well-being, social engagement and self-agency; neighbours; memories.

Taking these leads, a plan was developed for exploration with individuals using a prompt for open-ended and recorded discussion, in the form of a rotating circle, with eight segments, each containing a topic and prompts which the group-work had suggested. The 54 individual interviews that followed were founded on this new research tool, the Facets of Life (Figure 4.1).

As respondents turned the wheel to read the eight topics and their associated prompts, they could see at a glance the scope of enquiry and control the ordering of discussion by prioritising the topics which

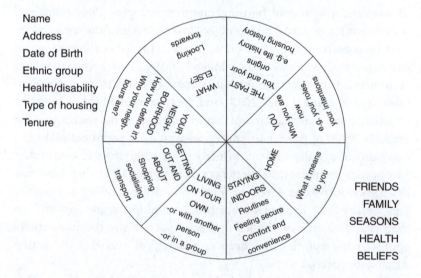

Name
Address
Date of Birth
Ethnic group
Health/disability
Type of housing
Tenure

FRIENDS
FAMILY
SEASONS
HEALTH
BELIEFS

Figure 4.1 Facets of life

interested them.[2] People were free to elaborate on or add topics or issues they thought relevant and to ignore whatever did not seem so important. The Wheel of Life seemed to enhance people's confidence in collaborating on these themes as they could anticipate the wider context and the ways their particular account might fit. We have already noted how previous approaches to measuring quality of life have tended to use sharply compartmentalised categories that do not allow the best representation of the mutability and continuity of life experience.[3] While based on what can be described as domains of life and living, in piloting and in subsequent data collection and analysis, the Wheel of Life seemed to permit expression of the inter-penetration of social and material aspects of environmental life as this might impact on identity. Moreover, it brings into focus the different and variable intensities that informants can attach to meanings they ascribe to each of the topics.

The academic context

Approaches to this research have been influenced by the multi-disciplinary fields of anthropology and material culture, geography, psychology, sociology and design. The theoretical background to the study is based in literature which covers: meanings of and attachment to home in later life; meanings and salience of neighbourhood; the social construction of space; quality of life in special living environments; person–environment interaction. Authors such as Soja (1989) and Massey (1994) have written influentially on space, time and identity. Bourdieu (1977) examined everyday life, notably how the environmental setting 'habitus' reveals the mechanism whereby ordinary practical experience evolves into habit and establishes custom and culture. Although he did not comment upon age-distinctive patterns, the fine-grained and subtle approach to the ordinary has provided one model for our approach to analysis. Design of domestic form and the 'social logic' that shapes customary internal configurations is addressed at another level in the theory put forward by Hillier and Hanson (1977). Others, notably Lefebvre (1991), have argued about the ways in which people at any age live and make sense of a changing world, and how past, present and future are constructed through spatial and temporal frames. Giddens (1984, 1991) discussed ontological security, recognising context as influential in supporting personal autonomy in everyday routines.

Within the field of gerontology an extensive body of literature has informed our approach. In a more explicitly structural and political connection, Townsend's (1981) argument for structured dependency reveals the importance of attachment to valued settings such as home, albeit as part of the segregation which Laws (1997) suggests society can impose on older people. Others have focused upon aspects of environment and ageing that concern meanings of home for older people (Sixsmith 1986, 1990; Gurney and Means 1993; Hockey 1999). Location has been considered across village life to urban neighbourhoods (Wenger 1984; Koskinen 2002; Scharf and Smith 2003) and research on movement and migration offers a context to informants' reflections on changing neighbourhoods (King et al. 2000).

The ecological model and ageing

The ecological model of Lawton and Nahemow (1973) introduced the concept of environmental press where the competence of individuals is considered alongside the immediate and wider environments in which they live. At the centre of the model was a level of adaptation where people are able to 'tune out' the environment and carry on without excess effort (Lawton 1980: 13). Such a state of equilibrium could, however, be disturbed by a number of shifts in or beyond the self, leaving the individual preoccupied and stressed. In later research Lawton suggested that the tension felt as a consequence of environmental press was not necessarily negative insofar as it stimulated a response to and engagement with environment (1983). The development of these ideas has been supported by further research on person–environment interaction in later life (Kahana 1982; Carp and Carp 1984; Carp 1987, 1994), and the ecological model continues to be debated and developed (Cvitkovich and Wister 2002). The material environment has also come to the fore through an accelerating interest in environmental design and assistive technologies (Kelly 2001; Peace and Holland 2001).

Spatiality in later life

Geographers in gerontology have proposed that appreciation and use of space tends to change in later years for individuals, groups and communities and our research is particularly influenced by Graham Rowles and Glenda Laws. In Rowles's seminal work *Prisoners of Space?* (1978), his theoretical perspective on the experience of older people in terms of space and place is based on the interdependency of four facets of experience that constitute a holistic framework encompassing an individual's environmental 'transactions'. First, *activity* covers habitual movement around the immediate setting and occasional more distant visits. Second, Rowles (1978: 171) observes how cognition or interest in particular spaces and places orders a hierarchy of significance from lived to 'beyond' space – *orientation*. Third, people's spatial experience can be expanded through *feelings*; emotional associations, for example, dread or elation can redefine place. Finally, more discursive facets of experience, often difficult to communicate, generate a fourth level of differentiated space termed *geographical fantasy* when places are experienced through recollection or imagination. Through placing this illuminating template around his data, Rowles shows how contextual cues such as objects and artefacts, rooms, streets, media, and to a lesser degree people, can stimulate geographical fantasy.

Rowles developed this schema by proposing the concept of 'insideness' (1983) which has three attributes: *physical insideness* – familiarity with the physical setting; *social insideness* – a degree of integration with the social fabric of community and possibly stressing links with the group culture of age peers; *autobiographical insideness* – arising out of a lifetime in particular environments. More recently he has argued for the dynamic transformation of space into place, to express the sense of 'being in place' (Rowles 1991, 2000; Rowles and Watkins 2003).

A further influence for this study has been Laws' elaboration on the spatiality of ageing from broader structural perspectives, seeing spaces and places as age graded and noting that 'youth is everywhere' (Laws 1994, 1997). The work of cultural geographers and sociologists on the spatiality of social life in later years (Zukin 1992; Pile and Thrift 1995) has been used by Laws to illustrate how over time space can be used to shape society's attitudes. Laws argues (1997: 93) for spatial dimensions of identity formation: 'Our identities are structured as much by material acts as they are by discursive practices.' The exercise of day-to-day influence and control, for example, through objects and routines, is however consequent upon capital resources and by extension, she says, to society and those structures that lie beyond the home. Laws's analysis extends to the domestic built environment as she suggests that the spatialities of age relations are also constructed through the separation of generations into different, increasingly remote households (1995). The experience of being old will, for example, vary according to household composition that entails people, spaces and place making.

Attachment to place

Attachment to place maintains the sense of self and identity across the years insofar as it engenders a degree of security as times change (Altman and Low 1992). The significance of place at different points in the life course has been considered by several authors (for example, Howell 1983; Marcus 1995; Zingmark et al. 1995). Whereas Bowlby (1953) saw attachment as related to early life experiences, Rubinstein and Parmelee (1992) see this as a life course phenomenon which involves place as lived and in memory. They take the argument further when they speak of spaces that can be adapted to support competence and those that can evolve to sustain internally held meanings of place.

Their model of place attachment in later life shows how any definition of place has to subsume time and space (Rubinstein and Parmelee 1992: 142). This is to be sensed in the energy and emotion that people bring to their accounts of spaces, building on objects or on reflections about places. The words used to describe spaces indicate significance and attachment, which may be 'strong or weak', 'positive or negative', 'narrow, wide or diffuse' (Rubinstein 1990). Rubinstein and Parmelee (1992) argue for three essential elements in understanding place attachment: geographic behaviour, identity and interdependence. The three elements span the collective – the meanings inherent to a given culture and shared by its members; and the individual – meanings derived from personal attitudes, beliefs and experiences. They make the case that place attachment is important to older people to keep the past alive, maintain constancy during times of change, and to support a sense of continued competence.

In earlier work Rubinstein (1989) also examined attachment through the microenvironment of home, elucidating connections between home environment (defined as the dwelling place and all the material objects it contains), and integration of home within the self.

An intensive analysis of a small group of older Americans yielded three classes of empirically derived processes: social-centred, person-centred and body-centred processes. In Rubinstein's view the recreation of shared (cultural) notions of correct standards and behaviour, which can take in each or all three processes, for example, the proper times and places for particular activities and so on, is a fundamental part of the mechanism that links person to place.

Key findings on a life of quality in old age

These approaches to understanding the environmental lives of older people represent a number of perspectives and disciplines, but they have one feature in common. They take holistic rather than segmented positions to draw out and analyse material on older people at home and in context. Furthermore, all take account of the ephemeral or intangible as they interpret data from the material world. It will be clear from the preliminary account of findings that follows how very influential these authors have been on our work. With the ideas of environmental press, insideness and socio-structural forces resonating, we now give voice to some of the older people in this study. First, from the heart of their familiar settings, then making observations on the external worlds which frame, inform and invigorate their domestic and inner lives, we aim to illuminate the mechanisms that link people to environment. We then consider how identity and quality appear in these accounts.

A first examination of the data, made up of 54 lengthy and often intense narratives, mostly recorded in the home setting, suggested that the older person–environment link could work at four significant levels: the home space; its material contents; gardens and yards; the immediate neighbourhood extending to the wider environment.

The home space

In the private space of their homes respondents had created complex worlds. Most were living in non-age related housing in mixed communities, alone or as couples. This generally meant that they had considerably more home space, even without outside storage and gardens, than people living in sheltered housing and residential care homes. In these special settings it should be said that limited space does not equate with simplified spatial experience. Many of them have distinct public areas for use in the daytime as part of care or support. The extent to which this kind of provision gives scope for fuller associative life varies and the proximity of others does not necessarily lead to meaningful contacts (Willcocks et al. 1987; Kellaher 2000). Moreover few, even those in ordinary domestic housing, considered that they had too much space. What was true for nearly all, whether they had a residential room or a large house, was the way they used their material and spatial resource to optimise social contacts that suited them. The couple speaking below show something of this:

> Well we have got two bedrooms, but over the years my husband, when we had a boy and a girl, so we are going back a long time, he built another room on the end of the bungalow, so it was a bedroom, so that made us three bedrooms. But gradually as they went, we changed it back to a dining room. But then with people coming to stay we still needed another room, so we have got a put-you-up bed. So the dining room can be turned into a bedroom. So we are back to the three bedrooms if we want ... when we have visitors.

This kind of account was very common as people described how they worked on their home environment to position themselves in relation to their networks of family and friends. Guest bedrooms were not an excessive indulgence, but necessary. Observations in this study showed that managing sleeping patterns which change with age can require an extra bedroom. Strengthening generational links seemed to be an important outcome to hospitality on the grandparents' territory, if not always on their terms. 'Extra' space could also be shared with adult children who could be helped when they ran into difficulties, such as family fractures and frictions.

Other 'excess' space was dedicated to obvious purposes such as storage, interests and hobbies. More widespread though less visible was the need for personal 'expansion' space. For some, especially among older men, this need was met by getting out and about, perhaps by car or public transport. Others needed to move around within the house. This was described as very purposeful, structured by habit and enacted spatially, mobilising and exercising all facets of the body. There were many versions of these ringings of the changes, each revolving around a unique set of domestic configurations, objects and intentions. Use of expansion space might be manifest in taking midday and evening meals in distinct places, or moving to different situations as the day and the light moved on. Most people, across the types of accommodation, mentioned a favourite or most frequented space at home, indicating that it was also crucial to move away from such an anchor point. These apparently mundane acts seemed to invigorate as they served to 'colonise' and differentiate spaces. Cumulatively, such habits build the structures, both spatial and temporal, through which social entity is made visible to self and others. Moreover, in choosing to access and quit spaces according to an individual interpretation of what is culturally appropriate, people sustain mastery and key into wider society.

Such movements and their transforming potential were more restricted for those in some special environments. The spaces to which residents of care homes or tenants/owners of sheltered housing have access may be different both in scale and configuration to the domestic. Issues of organisation, sharing and a decline in personal health also impinge. Where spatial allocations and layouts constrain, displays of a more complex self may be obstructed; for instance, the one-roomed residential space reflects a uni-dimensional persona so that the sense of identity becomes compromised. The abbreviated configurations of some sheltered housing units may similarly not conform to cultural norms. Psychological barriers emerge in some special settings when residents' access to parts of so-called 'public' space is limited (Kellaher 2000). This informant who speaks of life in a residential setting reveals dislocation from her customary understandings, giving an explanation she can only partly voice, and which may elude many in such situations:

> You see, my family said when I came 'You are to have lunch in the dining room', but one lady is so beyond it that she kept muttering and it made me depressed. So I had them [meals] in here ... It is very difficult ... it is so different – completely. This room in a way reminds me more of boarding school. But ... I mean they are so kind, you couldn't wish for anybody kinder ... No, I don't find it hard. I don't know what ... I miss home.

We can speculate that one aspect missed about home is the freedom to move around as desired, for instance, to take meals, between places that are appropriate – an option that appears to be foreclosed here. Since all informants made reference to the action of moving between points as a process having physical and psychological benefits, older people in settings or circumstances that curtail this process are seriously disadvantaged when it comes to using environment to sustain identity.[4] For the others, it was a habit they could continually refresh every time and from which they could draw confirmation as to who they were, because they were 'in place'.

The contents, objects and identity

Respondents frequently discussed the provenance of objects, that is large items of furniture and many smaller things such as ornaments, pictures and photographs. All these were available as cues and props to recount past and present, people and places; to recall previous dwellings and the people who lived there; and to speak of previous occupations, that is formally recognised employment as well as hidden work such as housework and incidental or episodic home work. Craft work of personal interests and images representing the achievements of family members were regularly volunteered for incorporation in accounts of home and how it supported these older people in being themselves. Photographs of grandchildren, often taken at degree ceremonies, were shown off. In terms of identity construction, these may be particularly significant since they look to a future and a past of skill and intelligence hitherto unrecognised and now realised. These descendants were shown as young people who were going to make it, occupationally, financially and socially. The implicit or unspoken commentary was sometimes that while the informant had not been so fortunate, now the kinship stock of health, looks, charm and cleverness could be seen and 'borrowed' by this oldest generation. The following enthusiastic example is not unusual:

> They keep bringing me photographs from the school and I don't know where to put them! [laughs] ... oh dear, and then they keep bringing them from the school you know. So then I put them altogether. They look and say, 'Well where is my photo nanny, you haven't got mine?'

This exchange shows again, how the social may be constructed and embellished from material things. With objects such as photographs the connection is clear, but people could also show things to which they claimed no particular attachment. These were said to be on display for others. Occasionally, an excess of gifts seemed to weigh heavily:

> I don't buy much. People buy me presents, people just give me things. All those vases I didn't buy them. I gave away some of these, and all those things ... a lot of people give them at Christmas. Mmm, there are too much things you can't even move, but I don't want to throw them away, you know. Sometimes I take them to the club and they sell them at the jumble sale. I couldn't throw them away. I wrap them up and give to who wants them. They gave me those at work when I retired.

This informant's view of 'clutter', along with things being 'minded' for others, shows how people allude to their networks of connections and the systems of obligation that link them.

Objects and the manner of their display can be seen as representing *self to self* (to remind, to reinforce selected aspects of personality); *self to others* (claims about personality and achievements); *others to self* (visual reminders of absent people, including changing images over time, for example, of grandchildren). While individual items were not on their own indispensable to the respondent's well-being, as a set, in many more ways than have been detailed above, they appear to underpin a sense of identity and ontological security. Such objects, and sometimes ephemera, are a focus for attachment, not through the relatively simple processes of ownership or possession, but through more complex mechanisms. These are made up of both incremental and fluctuating components, reflecting the continuity of identity across a lifetime and the adaptions and responses people have to make. Objects serve not just to reflect connections across time and place but also to reform them. Older people themselves and those who visit witness the objects, and recognise the significance of the identity they engender.

Gardens, patios, yards and window boxes

The boundaries of domestic and neighbourhood space are crucial. Our research begins to show the importance of the buffer space represented by the secluded garden, the paved patio or the unfenced grassed strip segregating the residential home from its surroundings:

> I do enjoy going out in the garden ... instead of sitting in front of the television, I always do the garden, mow the lawn, and the plants and everything. I like that.

73

The garden is a familiar, relatively controllable space that is unthrea-tening and yet permits encounter, however passive, with what might be the more risky neighbourhood. It nonetheless holds out a prospect of social exchange, for example, hearing the sounds of the neighbourhood can serve to define and confirm self. These features seem to become even more important if going out becomes problematic and the familiar home range contracts. This is shown in accounts of people who could get out only very occasionally and with help. What they could observe during daytime from their windows was drawn into who they were. Moreover, the garden or outdoor space calls out to be managed, cared for and controlled in the same way, but with other possibilities, as the internal domestic environment.

The natural world was important to many informants. There were those who could work and walk in their long-established garden, where plants were associated with the past and with particular people. There were others for whom pots and window boxes required continued care – and here pets should at least be mentioned. Even modest plantings offered a pretext for exchange and being in touch with the external world.

Proximate and wider neighbourhood

When it comes to settling in a new place, particularly in a care home, proximity and accessibility have often defined neighbourhood. Whilst there is an obvious point to be made about feeling familiar and secure about the place in which home is located and from which starting point older people may venture out, proximity, as Rowles has noted, can be displaced by more significant distant and even imagined places. At the same time, it has to be stressed that getting out somewhere is crucially important to older people. Environmental confidence may be challenged by changed health status or reactions to a resistant material environment. It can equally occur through a different set of factors and here again we may reflect on Rowles's biographical 'insideness'. A fracture in the social environment a close bereavement, for example, may lead to apprehension about a very familiar envir-onment, which is now perceived as threatening as the following account suggests:

> When my husband died I thought it was the end of the world. How am I ever going to … For three nights I sat up and cried, I couldn't even go into the bed.

Although the intimate domestic environment is implicated here, the respondent went on to describe how she was impelled to take action which involved getting out.

> I was so broken hearted … I used to cry here a lot on my own, and my sons used to come in and of course, I thought it was not fair to let them see me, they would only worry, and I thought to myself, 'I am going to get ill.' So I went out and joined a luncheon club, voluntary you know, and I joined things with my friends.

Her motivation in going to new places with new contacts was underpinned by concern for her adult sons and for the future of their relationships with her. The neighbourhood was a means rather than an end in itself. For others the neighbourhood may be more than this. A woman of 82 years illustrates several layers of the significance of neighbourhood, first of all the physical capacity to go out:

> I love my little bike. I never went very far, you know, but I still love it. My son says, 'Mum, you shouldn't be cycling at your age, I am going to smash up that bike' and I said, 'You don't dare!' I only go on the path to the church and up to the shops, you know. So it is exercise for me really, a good excuse.

Second, this woman engages with the immediate neighbourhood in a way that continues to define a facet of identity linked to a lifelong habit. The fact that her son challenges this and that she resists the challenge may be socially reinforcing in that, for the moment at least, they both are brought to an explicit acknowledgement of her identity as a woman who can go out, and in the way she chooses.

The character of the wider neighbourhood mattered to the older study participants in a number of ways, not least that it offered a wider context beyond that of the home. This proved to self and others that there was a social place to which they claimed belonging:

> I love it here, I mean I love my neighbours and I am at home here, I belong here. There is a sense of belonging. If I moved away there wouldn't be that sense of belonging. I think that is the word I would use.

Other more complex attributes associated with self and identity were derived from the character of the neighbourhood and wider environment. The degree of 'fit' between self-image and neighbourhood emerged as important. For example, respondents living in towns might express their original 'rural' identities through display of objects (pictures, pottery, photographs, plants). The same was true of older people who had arrived as migrants from other countries and cultures. The social heterogeneity of the neighbourhood, including the mix in terms of race/culture, age, wealth, class, and so on, mattered to these groups insofar as it allowed them scope for social transactions which set the scene for future help.

A high proportion of respondents' day-to-day contacts, especially in the case of those without cars but who went out regularly, were from the immediate half-mile radius neighbourhood. Such proximity carried an assurance that help could be at hand if necessary, more hopefully than expectantly. A few indicated that there came a stage in life, wherever one had ended up, when settling was called for since future assistance would rest upon being known locally and having connections. This level of pragmatism extended to a concern that the present neighbourhood should be supportive. People did not, however, discount the places they had moved from. An immigrant from India to Bedford said about the neighbourhood of settlement, 'My roots are there, but my branches are here.'

As already noted, no longer being able to go out independently marks a critical life stage. Without access to the wider context of the dwelling, the home itself becomes diminished as a source of identity. Continued capacity to engage with the 'other' is represented by neighbourhood in ways that the immediate domicile alone cannot demonstrate. It is also obvious that, whether simple or highly complex, the external environment of proximate neighbourhood can support as well as compromise mastery over movement and mobility that are crucial to self-esteem. For some older people, ageing is accompanied by an amplification of impact from micro environmental aspects of neighbourhood when, for instance, factors such as ground textures and formerly imperceptible changes in levels become problematic. Aspects of the external environment, previously managed without preoccupation, can turn into serious hazards, not only because they lead to physical injury when there are accidents, but also because confidence is eroded.

Environment and identity: time, place and space

Temporal and spatial aspects of environment were revealed through respondents' housing histories. In each of the three research sites we found people with lifelong, if intermittent, connections to the area. The present home frequently represented continuity or 'homecoming' that was location specific. For some the spatial continuity persisted despite change:

> I love it here. I really love it here. It has been my home sort of virtually all my life, because prior to the war I was at school and you know you didn't take much notice. But since then, I mean we started off with six of us here; mother and father, my sister and my two brothers. So, six of us lived here together and it was what you would call a real family home. And gradually ... well my sister went abroad and worked abroad all her life. And eventually my two brothers left of course, so there was just the three of us, mother, dad and I. And it was a family centre, you know, all the family kept in touch all the time.

For other respondents, the continuity offered by the location might become problematic, but as in this instance remained a point for connection:

> Well the thing about this street, when we were younger we used to know everyone that lived in all the houses, all by name, and in the Avenue as well, because my husband did window cleaning and he cleaned practically all the windows in the lane. And we got to know them because he did other jobs besides window cleaning ... and they were interested in us, and our family. But you don't get that now, people have died in this street, moved away, and there is a lot of people I don't know.

The conflation of time and place is inescapable in what these two people say about their home place. This was true of much that people had to say about their lives at home and in their neighbourhoods. The extent to which the personal identity of the respondents is vested in the status of their homes is complex. Here we have not touched upon the different tenures which link people to their dwellings, something that is likely to be patterned differently for future cohorts of older people. In presenting a little of what informants told us about their lives at home we suggest that there is a motivation common to these informants and this engenders the mechanism whereby environment and identity are linked.

Conclusion

The motivation we have witnessed relates to a need to maintain a life of quality, though it is not easy for these older people to spell out what this is or contains. The evidence from this research leads us to say that individuals judge which features of environment are significant at any given moment, mapping their needs and aspirations onto what is available and attainable in their physical and social environments. The correspondences are occasionally close, more often the fit is less than perfect and levels of environmental comfort may be compromised, but such strategic positioning continues throughout life. Lawton's case that people seek to 'tune out' the physical environment is supported by our findings. We would add that once the physical environment and its unwanted pressures is tuned out, the aim becomes the 'tuning in' to intimate, social and associative life, and to turn this to the desirable level of amplification for the individual. At such times a life of quality is registered. It is clear that subtle and strategic assessment in the context of a particular setting and circumstances is a constant requirement. We have found that older people engage in this kind of evaluation in the immediate term and in proximate environments as well as in the longer term, as when they weigh up the idea of moving to a new setting.

These individual, constantly reflexive and flexible calculations represent a level of engagement with the physical and social world which many have not associated with older people. The physical and material environment is acted upon and brought into play so that the person becomes as centrally placed as feasible in relation to their social network, however thin this may be. It is the fit between the nature and intensity of the connections a person has, and the level they want and can manage, that generates a life of more or less quality. Thus, a life of quality is one in which the sum of connections with foci outside the self – a few or many, constant or mutable – is sufficient to satisfy the particular individual.

The core finding from this study extends and integrates previous conceptions of the person–environment relationship in later life and develops Lawton's (1980) model of environmental press. The data show how people constantly generate, reinforce and dissolve connections with environment and that their range and intensity varies from person to person across the life course. There appears to be an essential comfort level for environmental connection that is to be maintained by creating a particular balance between self and society, reflexivity and reflectivity, inside and outside. Within their strategically chosen options, older people engage or disengage with particular activities, things, people and interests. Engagement levels can also shift, for example, after a change of environment or health status, as older people willingly or reluctantly reassess their ability to maintain the environmental status quo. Timing may be critical to the relative success of strategies for re-engagement; for example, in the case of relocation to residential care settings. Issues relevant for theory, policy making and practice, for example, privacy, inclusion and autonomy (Collopy 1988), might be considered afresh with the acknowledgement that even very frail older people aim to act strategically. Furthermore, their goal of connection with others and society is integral to their lives of quality.

Rather than quality of life being seen as a remote condition, to be drawn down and accessed by the fortunate individual, a life of quality emerges as a uniquely individual achievement, recognised as such by the principal protagonist and ideally endorsed by those who matter to that older person. Other people, family members, adult children, friends, neighbours and professionals may support the older person's version of quality. Sometimes, however, they may not be able to see and acknowledge the achievements of older people as they act within and upon environments habitually occupied or occasionally encountered. Even those very close and concerned do not share the perspective of the older person on the nature of the terrain, with its probabilities and hazards, the available options or more distant possibilities.

As an aspect of older people's housing need, neighbourhood has been relatively under-emphasised, yet it is clear that as people age the salience of neighbourhood increases. Our research suggests that policies on regeneration and development recognise how older people locate themselves somewhere close to the life of society and the lives of those who matter to them. The provisional finding that quality of life arises from social connection at the level and intensity desired by the older person has a familiarity, if not a banality, about it. Yet it may lead to a better appreciation of what older people aim for and realistically manoeuvre towards as they try to keep themselves, their inner and social identities going and experience a life of a certain quality.

Notes

1. Two sessions brought together people who had never met before. Most sessions were with pre-existing groups. Some groups were mixed gender, others women or men only. Two groups were people of a specific minority ethnic origin. Some groups were ethnically mixed, but most were made up of people of white British origin, ages ranged from 60 to 80 years. At this stage their housing tenure was not an issue but most groups included people who rented and people who owned their homes. Discussion, which was recorded, was generated through questions concerning housing, home and location.

2. This was a laminated card circle pinned onto an A3 backboard so that it could be rotated.

3. We also piloted the Southampton Self-Esteem Scale and the Philadelphia Geriatric Center Morale Scale concluding that the kind of data provided was covered more fluently by our new interview tool. The HOOP (Housing Options for Older People; Heywood et al. 1999) scheme proved time consuming and not sufficiently relevant since moving house was only one of many strategies our informants would consider. We eventually used the quality of life questions, inviting informants to complete the full HOOP as an optional extra to be posted back. To complement this data collection and to compare approaches, we used more structured questions to collect basic and supportive data about basic characteristics: health; financial status; housing satisfaction; HOOP Section 10 – well-being and quality of life. Housing history: summary of places where respondents had ever lived, reasons for moving; personality characteristics that might influence how the person interacted with their environment. Usual mobility range, accommodation layout – with interior, exterior, and location photographs. In a few cases it was not possible to collect the full suite of data but most sets were complete and all sets contained key data.

4. The importance of having enough space is confirmed in work undertaken by Hanson et al. (2003) for the UK Engineering and Physical Sciences Research Council.

5

Poverty and social exclusion – growing older in deprived urban neighbourhoods

Thomas Scharf, Chris Phillipson and Allison E. Smith

Introduction

The purpose of this chapter is to explore the experience of growing older from the perspective of older people who are potentially vulnerable to poverty and forms of social exclusion. Rising average pensioner incomes in recent years mask the widening gap between those older people who are better off and a substantial minority who continue to live in poverty (Darton and Strelitz 2003: 15). Evidence of growing income inequalities in Britain is matched by research that highlights the enduring nature of geographic inequalities (Hills 1995; Strelitz and Darton 2003: 91–103). In its most acute form, such area variations characterise the distribution of good health, and ultimately of life expectancy (DoH 1998a). In this chapter, we seek to link these themes together in order to develop understanding of dimensions of social inequality in later life and their impact on older people's wellbeing. This Growing Older Programme research examined the circumstances of older people living in areas of three English cities characterised by intense social deprivation.

The chapter is divided into five sections. First, we present an overview of existing research relating to poverty and social exclusion in old age, with particular emphasis placed on environmental determinants of exclusion. Second, we summarise the multidimensional approach used to measure poverty and social exclusion. Third, we outline the methods used in the empirical study. Fourth, we present key research findings in relation to the multiple risks of exclusion faced by older people in deprived urban areas. Finally, on the basis of a summary of these findings, we outline implications for public policy that arise from the research.

Poverty and social exclusion of older people

Questions about poverty and deprivation represent long-standing themes in research on ageing. Concern about the numbers of older people living in poverty found expression in the introduction of public pension systems in many European nations from the end of the nineteenth century. However, the subsequent development of modern welfare states did not always succeed in alleviating pensioner poverty. This was especially the case in the UK. In the 1950s and 1960s, researchers such as Cole and Utting (1962) and Townsend and Wedderburn (1965) identified older people as one of the largest groups living in poverty, with the widowed and the single elderly being especially vulnerable. This theme was given renewed emphasis with the rise of political economy perspectives on ageing from the late 1970s (Estes 1979; Walker 1980; Phillipson 1982). Here, poverty in old age was linked to the social construction of lifelong inequalities based around class, generation, gender and ethnicity (Minkler and Estes 1999). Townsend (1981) developed the idea of growing old as affected by a form of 'structured dependency', produced by the imposition of retirement, poverty and restricted social roles. Walker (1993), reviewing a large body of data, concluded that poverty in old age was primarily linked to individuals' low economic and social status preceding retirement and that the relatively low level of state benefits was of secondary importance.

This analysis was extended in the 1980s and 1990s with awareness of a widening of inequality between rich and poor of all ages (Hills 1998), and increasing inequalities developing among different groups of pensioners (Hancock and Weir 1994; Falkingham 1998). A key source of difference is between older people in receipt of an occupational pension and those who rely solely upon state benefits. While the average real incomes from occupational pensions rose by an estimated 152 per cent between 1979 and 1996–7, benefit incomes increased by just 39 per cent during this period (House of Commons 2003). The proportion of pensioners experiencing relative poverty, defined as earning less than half of average incomes, rose steadily through the 1980s and early 1990s. After housing costs, this proportion was 17 per cent in 1979, peaking at 30 per cent in 1998–9, before falling back to 25 per cent in 2001–2 (DWP 2003).

While social research continued to emphasise the persisting risk of poverty faced by many older people, neo-liberal social policy during the 1980s and early 1990s sought to limit debates about poverty. Income inequalities were perceived by government at this time as being the inevitable and legitimate outcome of a market-based economy. It is within this context that the notion of 'social exclusion' began to emerge as a theme in domestic social policy (Burchardt et al. 2002a: 3). Initially used by European Community policymakers as a means of developing a social agenda across the member states, the notion of exclusion increasingly provided the mechanism through which tradi-tional concerns about poverty could be raised. While there are clear overlaps between the dual concepts of poverty and social exclusion (Bhalla and Lapeyre 1997; Bauman 1998), the exclusion discourse sought to extend the poverty debate in important ways. In particular, social exclusion was regarded as a useful means of highlighting the social costs that can arise when individuals, families and communities become disengaged from wider society. Since the 1997 election, British social policy has been transformed by the Labour government's focus on tackling the causes and consequences of social exclusion (National Action Plan 2001).

However, 'social exclusion' (like poverty) remains a contested notion. Indeed, the flexibility of the term represents an important part of its appeal (Silver 1994: 536). The British government defines social exclusion as 'a shorthand term for what can happen when people or areas suffer from a combination of linked problems such as unem-ployment, poor skills, low incomes, poor housing, high crime, bad health and family breakdown' (Social Exclusion Unit 2001: 10). Other definitions highlight the multidimensionality of exclusion, suggesting that people can become excluded when particular institutional systems break down (Atkinson and Davoudi 2000). For example, Berghman (1997: 19) disaggregates the idea of exclusion, conceiving social exclusion in terms of the non-realisation of citizenship rights within

83

four key societal institutions – the democratic and legal system, the labour market, the welfare system, and the family and community system. Underlying several approaches to conceptualising social exclusion is also a concern with issues of place and space (Madanipour et al. 1998). This theme has been especially well represented in the work of researchers based at the LSE's Centre for the Analysis of Social Exclusion (Glennerster et al. 1999; Lupton and Power 2002: 118–40). The spatial dimension of exclusion is particularly important given the way in which neighbourhoods contribute to shaping the self-identities of those who reside in them. In this respect, Marcuse (1996) argues that the neighbourhood increasingly defines 'who a person is and where he or she belongs in society' (see also Chapter 4 this volume).

While the concept of social exclusion has become a central feature of both research and policy debates in recent years, to date these debates have focused most strongly on the needs of children, young adults and those of employment age (for example, Opportunity for All 2002; Hills et al. 2002). The absence of adequate data on the nature of poverty and exclusion experienced by older people (Howarth et al. 1999) further reflects the marginal position of this group in current debates about social exclusion (Scharf et al. 2001). Against this background, there are at least three difficulties that arise when seeking to apply the concept to the situation of older people. The first concerns the centrality of labour market participation as an indicator of social inclusion. Levitas (1998) identifies what she refers to as a 'Durkheimian conspiracy' lurking behind current social exclusion debates. The consequences of such an approach are social policies aimed at achieving cohesion through integration into occupational roles. The focus of exclusion debates on work and employment leaves unclear the position of older people who have permanently withdrawn from their occupational roles. This is especially relevant given that research in social gerontology has consistently highlighted the exclusionary impact of retirement on many older people (Phillipson 1998).

A second difficulty arises from an emphasis in exclusion discourse on the dynamic nature of social exclusion (Byrne 1999). Household panel studies show how people move in and out of poverty/exclusion as their circumstances change (Leisering and Walker 1998; Burchardt 2000; Burgess and Propper 2002), with the evidence suggesting that, as Perri 6 (1997: 6) asserts, 'most people get out of poverty'. For many younger people the boundaries of exclusion appear to be rather fluid. However, the situation of older people is likely to be rather different. For those prone to exclusion, its boundaries may be more rigid than would be the case for other groups. Thus, while exclusion from political activity or social interaction might represent an episodic characteristic of younger people's lives, older people may face additional difficulties in seeking to escape the enduring impact of such situations. Equally, older people who lack adequate material resources are unlikely to be able to 'get out of poverty' without considerable additional financial support from the state. This is a particular problem for those who live alone, with single pensioners – disproportionately women – representing one of the groups most likely to experience persistent low incomes (Walker 1981). Between 1997 and 2000, 20 per cent of single pensioners spent three or more years living in a household with below 60 per cent of median income (DWP 2003: 129; Table 7.9). Research on older people's experience of exclusion should consequently acknowledge the potential difficulties of achieving inclusion as a result of the relative stability of later life for many people.

A third problem concerns the neighbourhood dimension of exclusion (Scharf et al. 2002a). The local residential environment may represent a much more important aspect of exclusion for older people than for other age groups. On the one hand, older people tend to spend more time than younger people in their immediate neighbourhood. On the other, many older people have spent a substantial period of their lives in a particular neighbourhood, deriving a strong sense of emotional investment both in their home and in the surrounding community (Young and Willmott 1957; Phillipson et al. 2000). Indeed, Rowles (1978: 200) suggests that what he refers to as a 'selective intensification of feelings about spaces' might represent 'a universal strategy employed by older people to facilitate maintaining a sense of identity within a changing environment'. However, for older people living in rapidly changing urban communities it may prove difficult to maintain self-identity. This may apply to so-called 'zones of transition' marked by a rapid turnover of people and buildings, and to what Power (2000: 12) describes as 'non-viable' estates – those unpopular urban neighbourhoods characterised by low housing demand and subsequent abandonment of housing by all but the very poorest or least mobile residents.

A further element of neighbourhood exclusion that is especially relevant to the situation of older people concerns the infrastructure of their local community. Socially deprived neighbourhoods and the people who reside in them may be prone to what Gans (1972) refers to as 'institutional isolation' as services and agencies withdraw from areas judged to be economically marginal. The relative isolation of deprived areas in relation to both private and public sector institutions can raise acute problems for residents. Residents of disadvantaged neighbourhoods may even experience difficulty in accessing the most basic services, such as energy, food retailing, telephones and banking (Speak and Graham 2000). For older people with limited incomes or restricted mobility, the loss or absence of local services, including sub-post offices or affordable local shops, can be especially problematic, necessitating dependence upon others and/or the use of more costly means of transport. Inaccessibility of services might also reinforce an inhibition among some older people to use services. In this respect, Kempson and Whyley (1999) found that a considerable proportion of people aged 70 and over belong to a cash-only generation. Limited access to basic health and social care services or to public transport could represent further dimensions of older people's exclusion from key public and private sector institutions.

To summarise, research on social exclusion among older people needs to acknowledge traditional concerns with issues of poverty and deprivation. However, consideration should also be given to other dimensions of exclusion that are likely to be relevant to the situation of older people. In this respect, it is also important to explore forms of participation that reach beyond the labour market, the degree to which exclusion experienced by older people may be relatively static, and the high salience of the local residential setting in later life.

Measuring poverty and social exclusion

Moving from a broad conceptualisation of poverty and social exclusion to the empirical testing of these ideas represents a challenge for social research. The research we undertook for the Growing Older Programme built upon earlier work that operationalised social exclusion in a multidimensional way. For example, Burchardt et al. (2002b: 30–43) identify four domains of social exclusion that relate to the individual's ability to participate in what might be perceived as 'normal' social activities: consumption activity; production activity; political activity; social activity. A similar approach has been adopted by researchers engaged on the Joseph Rowntree Foundation's Survey of Poverty and Social Exclusion, albeit with different indicators of exclusion (Gordon et al. 2000: 54). Here, social exclusion is conceived of in terms of four dimensions: impoverishment; non-participation in the labour market; lack of access to basic services; exclusion from a range of social relations. This latter component is further subdivided into elements such as individuals' non-participation in common social activities, social isolation, a perceived lack of support in times of need, lack of civic engagement, and an inability to 'get out and about' (Bradshaw et al. 2000).

While the approach we adopted displays deliberate overlaps with these earlier studies, in its detail it seeks to accommodate factors judged particularly relevant to the circumstances of older people, and especially those living in deprived areas. Thus, we conceive of exclusion as encompassing five dimensions:

- exclusion from material resources
- exclusion from social relations
- exclusion from civic activities
- exclusion from basic services
- neighbourhood exclusion.

Each dimension has multiple components, chosen to reflect our conceptual understanding of exclusion in later life. For example, exclusion from material resources subsumes the dual components of (material) poverty and deprivation, while exclusion from basic services incorporates individuals' access to services both within and beyond the home. Ultimately the research sought to summarise each dimension of exclusion with reference to a single composite indicator. First, it is necessary to describe the empirical study which was undertaken to examine the degree to which older people in deprived areas experience poverty and social exclusion.

Methods

The first stage of the research involved selecting geographic locations in which to conduct a programme of research. Drawing on the 1998 Index of Local Deprivation (DETR 1998) – which at the time the research began represented the most recent measure of deprivation – Liverpool, Manchester and the London Borough of Newham were identified as the three most deprived English local authorities. To account for variation in relation to the spread and intensity of deprivation, the three most deprived electoral wards in each city were selected (Table 5.1). The study areas were Clubmoor, Granby and Pirrie in Liverpool; Cheetham, Longsight and Moss Side in Manchester; and Park, Plashet and St Stephens in Newham. While the selected study areas vary in relation to their proximity to the respective city centre, socio-economic structure and population profile, they share a range of characteristics associated with intense urban deprivation. This includes, for example, above average rates of unemployment, relatively poor housing conditions, a steady loss of services such as shops and banks, and a high incidence of crime (Social Exclusion Unit 1998). All nine wards were ranked among England's 50 most deprived wards in 1998.

Table 5.1 Study areas

Ward name	Local authority district	Ward's ranking on 1998 deprivation index
Granby	Liverpool	4
Clubmoor	Liverpool	7
Longsight	Manchester	16
Cheetham	Manchester	17
Pirrie	Liverpool	20
Moss Side	Manchester	38
Park	Newham	42
Plashet	Newham	46
St Stephens	Newham	50

Source: DETR (1998)

Second, in order to develop a fuller understanding of lay perspectives on such key themes as 'social exclusion' and 'quality of life', seven group discussions were conducted with older people. The groups were identified through contacts made by the researchers with relevant community groups. Three discussions were held in Newham, two in Liverpool, one in Manchester and, for the sake of comparison, one in a more affluent part of central England. Transcriptions of the taperecorded discussions informed subsequent phases of data collection.

Third, the research collected a range of primary data in two main phases. The first phase consisted of a detailed questionnaire survey of older people in the three cities. The purpose of the survey was to collect, first, socio-demographic data about the circumstances of older people living in deprived areas and, second, information relating to the themes of social exclusion, including:

- characteristics of poverty and its impact on daily life

- networks (including support networks) of older people

- patterns of support within the older population and with other social groups

- characteristics of social participation within deprived localities

- experiences of the urban environment in relation to services, crime, transportation and related issues.

Following two stages of piloting, trained interviewers conducted face-to-face interviews with 600 people aged 60 and over. Recruitment of participants occurred in two ways. A first group was randomly selected through local electoral registers using a coding classification that assigns people to age bands according to the likelihood that their first name belongs to a particular birth cohort. In this way 501 respondents were recruited (response rate – 42 per cent). A second group was recruited from the largest minority ethnic group in each electoral ward, drawing on relevant community organisations and researchers' local contacts. The aim was to generate a sufficiently large sample from each group to facilitate statistical analysis. Ninety-nine older people from four different minority groups (Black Caribbean, Indian, Pakistani, and Somali) were recruited. Interviews were undertaken in the language of respondents' choice by members of the research team, or by interviewers recruited from the relevant minority groups. Variation in the number of interviews with older people belonging to minority groups largely accounts for the different sample sizes in each study area. The number of respondents varied between 188 (Newham) and 206 (Liverpool and Manchester) in each city, and between 55 and 95 in each ward.

A second phase of data collection involved conducting semi-structured interviews with 130 people aged 60 and over. Ninety interviews were undertaken with people who had previously taken part in the survey, and had consented to be contacted again. Further interviews were undertaken with people belonging to populations identified through the survey as being particularly vulnerable to poverty and social exclusion. In this context, in-depth interviews were conducted with 20 older Somali people in Liverpool and 20 older Pakistani people in Manchester. These interviews explored such issues as older people's experiences of daily life, strategies for survival in urban areas, management of household finances, and the types of social relationships in which they were engaged. Largely for reasons of space, data from the in-depth interviews are not reported in this chapter (Scharf et al. 2002b).

Research findings

The intention in undertaking the empirical study was to generate data that would cast new light on the experience of ageing in deprived urban communities. In this respect, the research did not attempt to generate a sample that was representative of the older population of the UK as a whole. Nevertheless, it is useful to precede the presentation of research findings with a brief description of the sample with reference to the national picture (Table 5.2). In this respect, the survey sample does not differ greatly from that of the UK as a whole in relation to gender, especially at age 75 and above. Differences are more marked in terms of respondents' marital status. Compared with national samples, respondents in this survey were significantly less likely to be married or living as part of a couple. The survey sample is ethnically diverse, reflecting the population profile of socially disadvantaged urban neighbourhoods. Of respondents 70 per cent described themselves as white, 13 per cent as Black Caribbean, 7 per cent as Somali, 5 per cent

Table 5.2 Demographic characteristics of deprived area sample compared with UK sample

Sex	Deprived areas (60+)	GHS 1998 (60+)	Deprived areas (75+)	GHS 1998 (75+)
Male	41%	46%	37%	39%
Female	59%	54%	63%	61%
Marital status		**GHS 1998 (65+)**		**GHS 1998 (75+)**
Single	9%	6%	8%	5%
Married/living as a couple	42%	56%	27%	42%
Separated/divorced	10%	5%	6%	4%
Widowed	39%	35%	60%	48%

Source: GHS (Living in Britain) Tables 3.11, 5.2

as Pakistani, 4 per cent as Indian and 2 per cent as belonging to another ethnic group. Compared with national samples, survey respondents displayed significantly lower levels of owner occupation. Of respondents 58 per cent rented their homes, while 42 per cent were owner occupiers or in the process of purchasing their homes.

Exclusion from material resources

Turning to the different dimensions of social exclusion outlined above, the research first examined the material dimension of social exclusion. This was reflected in measures of deprivation and poverty. In relation to deprivation, the research built on the work of Evandrou (2000), whose 'index of multiple deprivation' comprises seven items considered especially important to older people (for example, central heating, use of a telephone, access to a car) (Box 5.1). The measure categorises people according to the degree of deprivation faced, ranging from no deprivation (where a person is not disadvantaged on any of the seven characteristics) to high deprivation (disadvantaged on at least five characteristics). The research found relatively high levels of deprivation among respondents (Table 5.3). The majority were classed as experiencing medium levels of deprivation, being disadvantaged on either three or four of the seven characteristics. Deprivation was

Box 5.1 Index of multiple deprivation

A person scores 1 for each of the following characteristics:

+ Lives in a household without central heating.

+ Lives in a household without a phone.

+ Lives in a household without a car.

+ Lives in local authority or housing association rented accommodation.

+ Lives in a household with more than one person per room.

+ Lives in a household where the head of the household receives income support.

+ Individual has no formal qualifications.

No deprivation: score 0, not disadvantaged on any of these characteristics.
Low deprivation: score 1–2, disadvantaged on one or two characteristics only.
Medium deprivation: score 3–4, disadvantaged on three or four characteristics.
High deprivation: score 5 or more, disadvantaged on at least five characteristics.

Source: Adapted from Evandrou (2000)

Table 5.3 Experience of multiple deprivation for 'white' older people in deprived areas of England and in Great Britain (%)

	Deprived areas 2001	Great Britain 1991–96*
No deprivation	3	30
Low deprivation	36	51
Medium deprivation	57	17
High deprivation	4	2
Total	100	100
	(n = 416)	(n = 28,080)

*Evandrou (2000)

especially pronounced for 3 per cent of respondents who fell into the category of high deprivation. Just 3 per cent were not disadvantaged on any of the characteristics, while 37 per cent experienced low levels of deprivation. Disadvantage was spread unevenly across the sample, with a heightened risk of multiple deprivation faced by older women, respondents aged 75 and over, those living alone, and older Pakistani and Somali people. Comparison of these findings with General Household Survey data reported by Evandrou (2000) suggests that older people in deprived communities experience a disproportionate and intense degree of multiple deprivation. In Evandrou's study, the bulk of white respondents were clustered towards the lower end of the deprivation spectrum. The research reported here reverses this, with almost three-fifths disadvantaged on at least three deprivation characteristics.

In relation to poverty, the research followed Gordon et al. (2000) by identifying as poor those respondents who said they were unable to afford what the majority of British people view as basic necessities. The research drew on the results of a national survey of the adult population, which highlighted items and social activities regarded by 50 per cent or more of people as being necessities of daily living (Gordon et al. 2000). Respondents in this study were presented with a similar list of 26 'socially perceived necessities'. Items included such basics as two meals a day, home contents insurance and the ability to replace worn-out furniture. People were asked to identify items that they didn't have or activities that they didn't do and to state whether they lacked the items because they didn't want them or couldn't afford them. As in the national survey, those lacking two or more items because they couldn't afford them were judged to be in poverty.

This research found 45 per cent of respondents to be living in poverty (Table 5.4). Forty per cent lacked none of the 26 items on the list of necessities for reasons of affordability, while a further 15 per cent lacked just one item. Some older people lacked and could not afford a substantial number of necessities, suggesting an intense degree of poverty. Seven per cent of respondents were unable to afford and were going without 11 or more of the items on the list. Taking only the 19 material items from the list of necessities, and adopting the same poverty threshold (lacking two or more items on the grounds of affordability), identifies 41 per cent of people as living in material

Table 5.4 Comparison of poverty rates for older people in socially deprived areas and the UK as a whole (%)

	Respondents unable to afford basic necessities	
	Deprived areas 2001	United Kingdom 1999*
Not in poverty (lacking 0–1 items)	55	79
In poverty (lacking 2 or more items)	45	21
Total	100 (n = 580)	100 (n = 405)

*Patsios (2001)

poverty (Table 5.5). The experience of poverty varied significantly according to respondents' ethnic background. Older people of Indian origin and those describing themselves as white were least likely to be in poverty, but for older people of Black Caribbean, Pakistani or Somali origin poverty was particularly pronounced. More than three-quarters of older Somali people (77 per cent) and two-thirds of older Pakistani people (67 per cent) were in poverty. By contrast, there was little variation in terms of gender or age. Older men were as likely to experience poverty as older women, and those aged 75 faced a similar risk of poverty as those aged 60 to 74 years.

Direct comparison of the survey findings with those of the national study shows older people in deprived areas of England to be at least twice as likely to experience poverty as those in Britain as a whole. The national survey classified 21 per cent of older people as poor (Patsios 2001), while the respective proportion in this study was 45 per cent.

The composite indicator of *exclusion from material resources* counts as materially excluded those older people who are both in material poverty and experiencing medium to high levels of deprivation. Combining the measures in this way focuses attention on those respondents who were likely to be experiencing greatest difficulty in making ends meet. This approach identified 31 per cent of respondents as being excluded from material resources (Table 5.6).

Table 5.5 Proportion of older people (aged 60 and over) excluded on different domains

Domain of social exclusion	Indicator of exclusion	% of respondents 'socially excluded' on indicator
Exclusion from material resources	In material poverty (lacks 2 or more socially perceived necessities on grounds of affordability)	41
	Multiple deprivation (deprived on 3 or more characteristics)	61
Exclusion from social relations	Social isolation (isolated on 2 or more characteristics)	20
	Loneliness (severely or very severely lonely)	16
	Unable to participate in 2 or more common activities	17
Exclusion from civic activities	Non-participation in civic activities	47
	Never attends meetings of religious or community organisations	24
Service exclusion	Has cut back on use of at least 3 of 4 basic services	14
	Not used 2 or more of 3 key services beyond the home	10
Neighbourhood exclusion	Expresses negative views about the neighbourhood	10
	Would feel very unsafe when out alone after dark	44

Table 5.6 Proportion of older people (aged 60 and over) experiencing exclusion on different domains

Domain of social exclusion	Composite indicator of exclusion	% of respondents excluded on domain
Exclusion from material resources	In material poverty and multiply deprived	31
Exclusion from social relations	Socially isolated or (very) severely lonely or unable to participate common social activities	41
Exclusion from civic activities	Non-participation in civic activities and never attends meetings of religious or community organizations	15
Service exclusion	Has cut back on use of basic services or has not used key services beyond the home	24
Neighbourhood exclusion	Expresses negative views about the neighbourhood and feels very unsafe when out alone after dark	21

Exclusion from social relations

Indicators of social isolation, loneliness and non-participation in common social activities were chosen to reflect different forms of exclusion from informal social relations. A *social isolation* measure was developed, drawing on individuals' availability of and the frequency of contacts with family, friends and neighbours (Box 5.2). In each case, isolation was judged to occur where individuals lacked relevant informal relationships, or where contacts with relevant members of the social network were infrequent (less than weekly). According to this measure, most older people appeared to be well integrated in informal relationships. Forty-four per cent of respondents had at least weekly

Box 5.2 Index of social isolation

A person scores 1 for each of the following characteristics:

♦ Has no relatives or children *or* sees a child or other relative less than once a week.

♦ Has no friends in neighbourhood *or* has a chat or does something with a friend less than once a week.

♦ Has a chat or does something with a neighbour less than once a week.

No isolation: score 0, not isolated on any of these characteristics.
Low isolation: score 1, isolated on one characteristic only.
Medium isolation: score 2, isolated on two characteristics.
High isolation: score 3, isolated on all three characteristics.

contact with family, friends and neighbours. A further 36 per cent experienced isolation on just one item, for example, lacking local friends. A minority of older people, however, were prone to social isolation. One-fifth of those taking part in the survey were judged to be isolated on two or three of the items included in the isolation measure (see Table 5.5).

Loneliness was measured using the De Jong Gierveld Loneliness Scale (de Jong Gierveld and Kamphuis 1985). The scale is based on responses to 11 items chosen to reflect the multidimensional nature of the loneliness concept. Adopting the cut-off points suggested by the scale's authors as a measure of the intensity of loneliness (de Jong Gierveld and van Tilburg 1999), 40 per cent of respondents were found to be not lonely (lonely on fewer than three of the 11 scale items), and 44 per cent could be described as moderately lonely. Sixteen per cent of those interviewed experienced either severe or very severe loneliness (lonely on nine or more scale items). Comparison with other studies that have used the same measurement instrument (de Jong Gierveld and van Tilburg 1999), and with research using different measures (Victor et al. 2000), suggests that older people in deprived areas experience a heightened risk of loneliness. This appears to correspond with earlier research conducted in the socially deprived inner London Borough of Hackney, where 16 per cent of older respondents were reported to be 'often' or 'very' lonely (Bowling et al. 1991).

Non-participation in common social activities is an indicator derived from the poverty measure outlined above (Gordon et al. 2000: 59f.). It encompasses seven activities perceived as necessities by a majority of the adult population. Almost two-thirds of respondents (65 per cent) were not excluded from any of these activities on the grounds of lack of affordability, and 18 per cent were excluded from just one activity. However, 17 per cent lacked and could not afford to participate in two or more common activities.

The summary indicator of *exclusion from social relations* recognises the relevance of each of the three forms of exclusion measured as representing important dimensions of exclusion from informal social relationships. In this regard, individuals were judged to be excluded if they experienced medium or high levels of social isolation, were (very) severely lonely, or were unable to participate in two or more common activities on the grounds of lack of income. While the majority of older people in deprived areas were not prone to this type of exclusion, just over two-fifths (41 per cent) were identified as excluded from social relations (see Table 5.4).

Exclusion from civic activities

Two measures assessed the degree to which older people were engaged in civic activities. First, respondents were asked whether they attended religious meetings or meetings of community groups. Forty-two per cent attended religious meetings at least once a year, and 33 per cent attended meetings of community groups. The remaining group, representing almost half of respondents (47 per cent), never attended either type of meeting (see Table 5.5).

Second, respondents were presented with a list of 11 civic activities and asked whether they had undertaken any of the stated activities in the three years preceding interview. The list encompassed a broad range of activities, chosen to reflect different types of civic engagement. Included in the list were activities such as writing a letter to the editor of a newspaper and taking part in fundraising drives. The most commonly observed civic activity was voting, with 68 per cent having voted in the previous general election and 66 per cent in the last local election. Taking all 11 activities together, we found that the great majority of respondents were actively engaged in at least some type of civic activity. Seventy-six per cent had undertaken at least one of the listed activities in the stated period. The remaining 24 per cent had not participated in any of the activities.

Respondents who did not participate in meetings of religious or community groups and who did not take part in any type of civic activity in the three years preceding interview were judged to be *excluded from civic activities*. Adopting this approach, the overwhelming majority of older people (85 per cent) in deprived areas participated in some form of civic activity. However, 15 per cent of older people were identified as being excluded on this indicator (see Table 5.6).

Exclusion from basic services

Access to basic services becomes increasingly important in later life, especially for people with restricted mobility or poor health. As suggested earlier, there is also evidence of particular difficulties faced by residents in deprived urban communities in accessing services. In this context, the research sought information about respondents' access to and use of a range of services both within and beyond the home.

In the home, the overwhelming majority of older people had access to basic utilities (gas, electricity, water, telephone). However, not all respondents made full use of these utilities, and a significant minority cut back on using such services in order to make ends meet. Respondents were asked whether in the previous five years they had used less water, gas or electricity or had used the telephone less often in order to save money. Just over three-quarters (76 per cent) had not cut back on any of the services. However, a small minority had experience of cutting back on most services. 14 per cent had used less of three or four of the listed basic services (see Table 5.5).

Beyond the home, an indicator of service exclusion was derived from the non-usage in the year preceding interview of three key services judged to be particularly important to older people. These services – a post office, a chemist, and a bus service – were selected from a longer list of services and amenities. The overwhelming majority of older people in this study had made use of such services. While 72 per cent of respondents had used each of the three services at least once in the previous year, a further 18 per cent had used two of the services. The remaining 10 per cent had failed to use at least two of the three services.

The measure of exclusion from basic services seeks to combine the two indicators outlined above. We judge as *service excluded* those respondents who had used less of three or four services in the home in order to save money, or who had not used two or more key services outside the home. This applied to 24 per cent of older people in deprived areas (see Table 5.6).

Neighbourhood exclusion

The final dimension of social exclusion addressed in this research seeks to reflect the distinctive contribution of environmental factors to exclusion. As such, it provides an indirect measure of the neighbourhood's impact on respondents' self-identities. The research addressed the dimension of neighbourhood exclusion by examining individuals' perceptions of their neighbourhoods, and their feelings of security in the neighbourhood.

Older people's perceptions of their local neighbourhood were measured through a range of separate questions. In terms of exclusion, we were particularly interested in those people whose responses reflected the greatest degree of disenchantment with the neighbourhood. For example, respondents were asked first whether there was anything that they liked about their neighbourhood. This was followed by a similar question relating to dislikes. Combining responses to these two questions, we identified a small group of older people, amounting to just under one-fifth (18 per cent), who only expressed dislikes about the neighbourhood. Another question asked people how satisfied they were with their neighbourhood. This showed one in ten respondents to be 'very dissatisfied' with their neighbourhood. Finally, 13 per cent of those taking part in the research strongly disagreed with the statement 'this neighbourhood is a good place to grow old in'. To identify those older people with the most negative perceptions about their neighbourhood, and potentially finding it difficult to maintain a sense of identity in a changing environment, we combined people's responses to the three items. While the overwhelming majority of older people did not hold extremely negative views about their neighbourhood, 10 per cent of respondents expressed such views in relation to at least two of the three questions (see Table 5.5).

The degree to which older people feel secure when leaving the home after dark provides a further indicator of neighbourhood exclusion.

Those who regard their neighbourhood as unsafe or a place where they might be vulnerable to crime may be restricted in their ability to participate in important social roles. In this research, where many older people had personal experience of crime (Scharf et al. 2002b), it is not surprising that relatively few respondents would feel safe when leaving the home after dark. Just 7 per cent suggested that they would feel 'very safe'. By contrast, 44 per cent reported that they would feel 'very unsafe' under these circumstances.

The composite indicator of *neighbourhood exclusion* counts as excluded those individuals who expressed negative views about the neighbourhood in relation to at least two of the three questions outlined above, and who also reported that they would feel very unsafe in their neighbourhood after dark. Almost four-fifths of those questioned (79 per cent) were 'included' according to this particular measure. However, the remaining 21 per cent of respondents could be classed as excluded from their local neighbourhood (see Table 5.6).

The experience of multiple exclusion

Summarising the findings so far, it is evident that significant numbers of older people in deprived urban areas appear prone to different dimensions of social exclusion. Exclusion from social relations was the most common of the five types of exclusion identified, affecting around two-fifths of older people. Just under one-third experienced exclusion from material resources. Nearly a quarter were excluded from basic services, and just over one-fifth experienced neighbourhood exclusion. Around one in seven was excluded from participation in civic activities. Drawing these findings together, the research reveals the degree to which older people in deprived urban areas may be prone to one or more forms of social exclusion. A considerable proportion of respondents were found to experience at least one type of exclusion. In this regard, the study population divides into three categories (Table 5.7):

* The first group – the 'included' – comprising 30 per cent of respondents, were not excluded on any of the five domains.

* A second group – the 'vulnerable' – representing 31 per cent of the sample, experienced exclusion on a single domain.

♦ The final group – the 'excluded' – was numerically the largest, comprising almost two-fifths of respondents (39 per cent) who were prone to the cumulative impact of multiple forms of exclusion.

Table 5.7 Older people (aged 60 and over) experiencing multiple forms of exclusion

	%	(n)
Not excluded	30	179
Excluded on one domain	31	189
Excluded on two or more domains	39	232
Total	100	600

The experience of multiple exclusion was significantly linked to age and ethnicity. People aged 75 and over were more likely to be multiply excluded than those aged 60 to 74 years. Respondents of Indian and Black Caribbean origin were much less likely to experience exclusion than Somali and Pakistani older people. Four out of five Somali respondents (80 per cent) and just over half of Pakistani respondents (52 per cent) were excluded on two or more domains. By contrast, multiple exclusion did not vary significantly according to gender. In relation to geography, and reflecting in part the ethnic background of local residents, vulnerability to exclusion varied significantly between electoral wards. Multiple exclusion was most pronounced in Granby (Liverpool) where just 15 per cent of respondents were not excluded on any of the five domains, and 54 per cent were prone to at least two types of exclusion. This contrasts with Pirrie (also in Liverpool), where 52 per cent of respondents were not excluded on any domain, and 14 per cent experienced multiple exclusion.

The complex nature of social exclusion is reflected in analysis of the relationships between its constituent domains (Table 5.8). Of respondents who were excluded on the material dimension, 58 per cent were also excluded from social relations, 20 per cent from civic activities, and 33 per cent from basic services. Such findings underline the important role of poverty and deprivation in limiting older people's ability to fulfil key social roles. Exclusion from social relations was further related to exclusion from basic services and neighbourhood exclusion.

Table 5.8 The relationship between different domains of social exclusion

| | % of respondents excluded in relation to | | | | |
	Material resources	Social relations	Civic activities	Services	Neighbourhood
% also excluded in relation to:					
Material resources	–	43**	42*	43**	33
Social relations	58**	–	49	58**	55**
Civic activities	20*	18	–	20	15
Services	33**	34**	32	–	24
Neighbourhood	22	28**	21	21	–

*$p>0.05$; **$p>0.005$

In this regard, there is evidence of a neighbourhood impact on individuals' ability to engage in social roles. Older people who feel cut off from their surroundings are more likely to experience limitations in their informal relationships than those who perceive their neighbourhood more favourably. Exclusion from civic activities and neighbourhood exclusion were most likely to be independent of other forms of exclusion.

Social exclusion and quality of life

A focus of this research has been to explore interactions between social exclusion and quality of life for older people living in socially deprived urban areas. Having shown that older people in such neighbourhoods are prone to different types of exclusion, and that many are vulnerable to multiple forms of exclusion, the question arises of the degree to which this impacts upon quality of life. Elsewhere the research has shown the existence of a close relationship between three widely used standard measures of quality of life, and that a single-item measure which invites respondents to assess their own quality of life can offer an effective means of measuring subjective well-being (Smith et al. 2003). Cross-tabulation of the summary social exclusion and life quality variables shows that older people who rate their quality of life as 'good' or 'very good' are significantly less likely to experience social exclusion

Table 5.9 Relationship between quality of life and the experience of multiple forms of exclusion for older people (aged 60 and over)

Self-reported quality of life	Not excluded %	Excluded on one domain %	Excluded on two or more domains %	(n)
Very good	47	37	15	78
Good	37	36	27	267
Neither good nor poor	20	29	51	146
Poor	12	23	65	69
Very poor	6	0	94	18
All	30	32	38	578

than those rating their life quality as poor or very poor (Table 5.9). Put another way, the research suggests that social exclusion is closely associated with a diminished quality of life.

Conclusion

Implications for research and policy

From the conceptual discussion and the range of data presented, it is possible to make a number of observations about the nature of social exclusion and the way in which it affects older people in deprived areas of England. Most importantly, we have been able to demonstrate that older people in these areas face multiple risks of exclusion. Using a measure that reflects the multidimensionality of social exclusion in relation to the situation of older people, it was established that seven out of ten respondents could be classed as excluded in relation to at least one aspect of their lives. For almost two-fifths, the experience of exclusion in one area was compounded by vulnerability to additional types of exclusion. The risk of being affected by multiple forms of social exclusion was greatest for those in the oldest age group (75 and over), and for those belonging to some minority ethnic groups. The research also points to the existence of connections between the different domains of exclusion. In particular, there was a strong relationship between exclusion from social relations and exclusion from material resources. This tends to confirm the findings of earlier studies that emphasise the ways in which poverty and deprivation can combine to restrict participation in a range of informal social relationships (Townsend 1979; Mack and Lansley 1985; Gordon et al. 2000).

The research presented in this chapter also highlights the importance of paying attention to environmental influences on ageing. Where comparable data are available, it is evident that older people in deprived urban areas appear to be more vulnerable to the experience of different forms of social exclusion than those living in the UK as a whole. This was shown, for example, with reference to the risks of poverty and multiple deprivation, and loneliness. It will be important to conduct similar studies in other types of geographic location in order to identify the full extent of the spatial divide that marks old age in Britain.

Finally, this research presents important challenges to policymakers and practitioners involved in urban regeneration initiatives (Scharf et al. 2002b). First, the research highlights the importance of informal social relationships in older people's daily lives. Many older people like to stop and chat to people in the street, or visit family, friends and neighbours in their homes. In deprived areas there may be a range of physical and psychological barriers that prevent older people from engaging in such relationships. Urban regeneration programmes typically invest large sums in altering the physical environment of deprived areas, but they can also play a role in creating public and private spaces that could encourage the development of informal social relationships. Housing schemes with pleasant and secure public spaces, shopping areas that provide places to sit, and community centres are important in this context. Measures that reduce neighbourhood crime are likely to have a positive impact on older people's social integration by removing some of the psychological barriers that inhibit their participation in a range of outdoor activities.

Second, there is the issue of older people's involvement in civic activities. Community engagement represents a route by which individuals can remain valued and effective. It may also rebound on older people's mental and physical health. This research shows that most older people in deprived areas already display some degree of commitment to public involvement. Only 15 per cent were not engaged in any type of civic activity. This suggests that there is considerable potential for increasing older people's participation in local decision making, but the characteristics of social exclusion may limit such activities. Material insecurity, low levels of literacy, language barriers, lack of self-confidence, and a perceived vulnerability to crime are likely to prevent some people from engaging more fully in their communities. Policymakers and planners can help to overcome such barriers by actively seeking the involvement of potentially vulnerable groups of older people in different stages of decision making.

Finally, the research highlights the overriding importance to older people in deprived areas of basic services. Local post offices, health centres, chemists and public transport are felt to be essential by most older people. It is important that public policy recognises the need to maintain access to a good service infrastructure in deprived urban neighbourhoods. Such areas continue to be highly vulnerable to the withdrawal of both public and commercial services. Older people who are already disadvantaged in terms of poverty or ill health are disproportionately affected by the loss of services such as a local post office or shops. As a result, consideration should be given at an early stage to the likely impact on older people of decisions to withdraw services from deprived neighbourhoods. Policies that can maintain the service infrastructure of such areas will not only benefit older people, but are also likely to benefit the community as a whole.

Acknowledgements

The research was undertaken with the financial support of the Economic and Social Research Council under its Growing Older Programme (L480254022). The authors wish to acknowledge the contribution of Paul Kingston to the research reported here.

6

Loneliness in later life

Christina R. Victor, Sasha J. Scambler, John Bond and Ann Bowling

Introduction

Social factors, especially social engagement and participation, are key dimensions in defining and enhancing quality of life in old age (and probably at earlier phases in the life course). Indeed Rowe and Kahn (1997) suggest that in advanced old age social factors are more important than biological or genetic factors. They argue that engagement with life, as defined by the maintenance of social relationships and 'productive activities', is one of the three key factors for 'successful ageing'. Given the theoretical and empirical importance ascribed to social engagement for the quality of life of older people, we can infer that the absence of social relationships and engagement or dissatisfaction with the extent or quality of such relationships or levels of engagement will have a detrimental influence upon the quality of life of older people. However, measuring the complex web of relationships that define the social world of older people can be problematic. Hence loneliness is often used as an exemplar of social engagement because it is a factor that is seen as being integral to quality of life in old age (Gibson 2001).

The interest in and recognition of the importance of the 'social world' or social context upon the experience of ageing is not new. In Britain these issues were first described and discussed in the classic studies of Sheldon (1948) and Townsend (1957) who investigated the social relationships of older people both locally (Sheldon 1948 and Townsend 1957) and nationally/internationally (Townsend 1968). All of these studies examined the nature and extent of social engagement among older people. Their focus was upon measuring the extent of loneliness and social isolation among older people and identifying risk factors for loneliness/isolation. The (implicit) intention was the development of screening tools and interventions by which loneliness could be identified and 'ameliorated' and social engagement promoted and enhanced as a means of promoting quality of life in old age. This was a policy-related research agenda not too dissimilar to the GO programme with its emphasis upon identifying the factors that define and enhance quality of life in old age.

Theoretical and conceptual issues

Loneliness as a concept is theoretically and conceptually complex (see de Jong Gierveld 1999; Victor et al. 2000) and is a term often used in empirical research in a vague and ill-defined manner. At the most simplistic level loneliness is concerned with how individuals evaluate their overall social network and their levels of social interaction and engagement. Loneliness describes the state in which there is a deficit between the individual's actual and desired level of social engagement (Hazan 1980). Hence this is an inherently 'relative' concept – it is concerned with how people feel about their social world rather than the 'objective reality'. As such loneliness needs to be distinguished from three related but not coterminous concepts. These are being alone/aloneness (time spent alone), living alone (simply a description of the household arrangements) and social isolation (which refers to the level of integration of individuals (and groups) into the wider social environment). Clearly these four different concepts share some commonality although the precise degree of overlap is unclear and the terms should not be used interchangeably (Victor et al. 2000).

Theoretical perspectives on loneliness come from a variety of different disciplines. However the major conceptualisations of loneliness are usually characterised by the identification of two distinct forms of the condition. Witzelben (1968) distinguishes how primary or existential loneliness is conceptualised as something that is inborn in all of us, the notion of being 'alone' in the world, and secondary loneliness, resulting from the loss of someone (or something) that is important to the individual. Weiss (1973) offers another typology of loneliness: emotional and social. Emotional loneliness is defined by the lack of close, intense personal relationships, whereas social loneliness is conceptualised in terms of a lack of overall social engagement and a limited social network. Another framework suggests a distinction between loneliness that derives from the personality or temperament of the individual and that which derives from the situation or circumstances that individuals find themselves in such as bereavement or the ill health of a spouse. Typically theories of loneliness focus upon the individual and posit micro-level factors in understanding the nature of loneliness. Few have taken an explicitly sociological focus which has tried to incorporate macro-level social forces.

Issues of measurement

The lack of consistency of conceptualisation is reflected in the varying ways that loneliness is defined and measured. It is often defined and measured as the subjective counterpart to the more 'objective' concept of social isolation (Bowling et al. 1991), or the antithesis to social support (Jones et al. 1982). Measuring such a nebulous, but vital, concept is problematic and studies rarely make explicit the theoretical conceptualisation that underpins the work. Two main approaches towards the empirical measurement of loneliness may be identified in the research concerned with older people; the use of single question self-rating scales as pioneered by Sheldon (1948) and the development of specialised scales, such as the UCLA loneliness scale (Russell 1996) or de Jong Gierveld, (1999) scales.

In Britain most research with older people has relied upon 'simple' self-report Likert scale type questions and asked respondents to rate their feelings of loneliness on a scale from never to always, with varying gradations of response ranging from three to seven point scales. Such measures have no explicit theoretical underpinning with a particular conceptualisation of loneliness and may fail to differentiate different types of loneliness that may be experienced by older people, although Sheldon (1948) clearly had an implicit view of loneliness as being largely secondary in nature, that is the response of individuals to specific external social circumstances. Clearly such measures are not without their methodological limitations. They are explicit and unambiguous in asking directly about loneliness, often in direct interview settings. The overt nature of the question offers the clear potential for a clash between the 'public' and 'private' faces of the individual older person. Privately the older person may feel lonely but might not wish to 'admit' this to an interviewer for fear of compromising their public persona as a competent individual and attracting the social stigma attached to such negatively defined groups. Additionally such measures presuppose a common understanding of the term 'lonely' which may (or may not) be present among older people.

A variety of specialist scales has been developed to address the potential shortcomings in the standard 'self-report' measures. Rather than relying upon the evaluation by individuals of their own experience, these measures use largely indirect questions to determine both the prevalence and intensity or severity of loneliness. Such measures have been developed for use with all groups in Europe (de Jong Gierveld) and the USA or specifically for older people such as the scale devised by Wenger (1984). Typically such measures ask about satisfaction with levels of contact with family and friends and availability of confidants. Such measures are not without limitations. They ask 'indirectly' about loneliness and are underpinned by a presumption that it is more revealing to ask indirectly about this emotive topic. It has been suggested that for older people self-report scales are most appropriate (Holmen and Furukawa 2002).

Limitations of previous research

Although the landmark studies of Sheldon, Townsend and Tunstall are exemplars of social research of their time and provide valuable insights into the experience of old age, they are now rather 'dated' and were undertaken within a profoundly different social context. Sheldon undertook his fieldwork in the immediate post-World War II period, while Townsend and Tunstall's work was undertaken in the late 1950s and early 1960s. Much has changed in British society since, as the population has become more diverse. For older people a key factor that has undergone remarkable change over this period is in the percentage of people living alone. When Sheldon (1948) undertook his fieldwork in Wolverhampton, approximately 4 to 10 per cent of people aged 60 to 65 and over lived alone, compared with 36 per cent in 2001. Given that living alone has consistently been identified as a 'risk factor' for loneliness, we might expect that contemporary cohorts of elders would show greatly increased levels of loneliness. In addition many of the studies used as the basis of estimating the prevalence of loneliness are focused in specific localities such as London (Townsend 1957), North Wales (Wenger et al. 1996), South Wales (Jones et al. 1982), Sheffield (Qureshi and Walker 1989). There is a clear need for a contemporary study based upon a nationally representative sample to build upon the work of Townsend (1968) and Hunt (1978). Since many of the initial studies which established the 'risk factors' for loneliness there has been considerable development of social science methods. This means that we can now use multivariate statistical modelling to establish the independent relationships between individual risk factors and loneliness. Hence we can determine if the relationships between gender, age, living alone and widowhood are independently associated with loneliness or whether, for example, only widowhood is linked with loneliness and the other relationships are the result of confounding.

Aims of the project

Our project set out to investigate the relationship between loneliness, social isolation and living alone and to identify factors protective against isolation and loneliness among a contemporary nationally representative cohort of older people living in the community. In particular we sought to achieve five key objectives:

◆ the description of contemporary 'peer group' patterns of loneliness and isolation among older people living in the community

◆ to contribute to policy and practice by identifying the factors, resources and coping mechanisms that protect and place older people 'at risk' from experiencing loneliness and isolation

◆ to investigate preceding cohort patterns of loneliness by making direct comparisons of our results with the classic British studies of Sheldon (1948), Townsend (1957, 1968) and Tunstall (1966)

◆ to examine age-related patterns of loneliness by placing current levels of loneliness and isolation within a life course perspective

◆ to investigate the relationship between loneliness and social isolation and living alone for older people.

In this chapter we focus upon peer group, age-related and preceding cohort patterns of loneliness.

Methods

The study captured data from two main sources: a quantitative survey of loneliness and social participation and an in-depth qualitative study of a purposive sample of participants identified from the initial survey. Given the explicit comparative nature of one arm of the project, decisions concerning the design of the qualitative study were influenced by this requirement.

The interview survey

The interview survey was undertaken to achieve the objectives concerned with prevalence and patterns of loneliness and isolation among older people. The survey was conducted as part of the Office for National Statistics Omnibus Survey. This is a face-to-face interview conducted with approximately 1000 adults aged 16+ in their own homes which is undertaken monthly (or bi-monthly depending upon demand). The Omnibus Survey selects 30 addresses randomly from a sample of 100 postal sectors across Great Britain and from this provides a relatively large, nationally based, randomly selected, broadly representative sample of the adult population resident in the community.

Respondents aged 65 and over participating in the Omnibus Survey were invited to participate in our Quality of Life module that was administered at a second interview. This was a collaborative venture between ourselves and two other research groups (at University College London and Bristol University) that added value to all three studies. The use of ages 65 years and over to define our target population, and the restriction of the sample to those living in the community, was to secure the comparability of our data with our index surveys. To control for seasonal effects and to generate a sample of sufficient statistical power, we were aiming for a sample of approximately 1000 respondents, four sweeps of the module were conducted at quarterly intervals. All respondents aged 65 and over interviewed for the April, September, November 2000 and January 2001 Omnibus Surveys were invited to participate in our Quality of Life survey and those who agreed were reinterviewed two months after the initial contact.

As one of the key objectives of the project was to make direct comparison with the 'classic' UK studies of loneliness/isolation, thereby enabling some examination of preceding cohort patterns of loneliness, this informed our selection of topics and measures. To replicate the work of Tunstall and colleagues we measured loneliness using a self-rating scale. This invited participants to classify their levels of loneliness on a four-point scale ranging from often to never. Age-related loneliness was measured using a question inviting respondents to compare current levels of loneliness with that of a decade earlier and evaluate themselves as 'better', 'worse' or unchanged. Standard demographic and health data were also collected along with details of social activities and contacts with family, friends and neighbours (see Bowling et al. 2002 and Ayis et al. 2003 for further details of the survey and range of data collected).

By linking the responses to the current evaluation of loneliness and changes over the past ten years, we were able to identify our theoretically derived subgroups of loneliness in later life. In particular we wished to start to explore the distinction between the existential or temperamentally lonely group, for whom loneliness in later life represented a continuation of a previously established pattern of life and those for whom loneliness may be the result of changes in the social environment (secondary loneliness) and as such was a 'new' or recent experience. Using potential responses to our two questions we developed the following typology:

1. The temperamental/lifelong lonely group was defined as those who reported that they were always/often lonely and also reported an unchanged level of loneliness.

2. Those who were often/always lonely and for whom this represented an increased level of loneliness were defined as our 'late onset' group and we suggest that this group may be those for whom loneliness develops as a response to a major dislocation in their social/ emotional context.

3. Those who reported that they were sometimes/never lonely and that this was an improvement on the previous decade were defined as our 'improvers' group. Although not derived theoretically this

113

group may well identify those for whom secondary loneliness was decreasing as they adapted to their changed circumstances.

4. Finally there was the group who reported that they were never lonely and this was unchanged. These were defined as our never lonely group.

Analysis strategy

Our strategy was to test for univariate patterns of association between loneliness and specific risk factors in a preliminary analysis. Individual 'risk factors' were grouped into five categories: socio-demographic factors, health resources, material resources, social resources and social network. Ordered logistic regression was used to test the independence of association with our outcome variable (loneliness).

The qualitative study

The qualitative study consisted of 44 in-depth, semi-structured interviews with 18 men and 27 women aged between 65 and 90 selected from participants in the quantitative survey. Participants were initially selected from five areas of the country to replicate the types of areas included in the study by Tunstall. These areas were the South Coast (a typical retirement area), East Anglia and the South West (rural areas), the East Midlands and the North-East (urban, industrial areas). Following the pilot study, two other areas were included – London (a metropolitan area) and Surrey (an affluent commuter belt). An interview topic guide was followed incorporating the ways in which people spent their time, the people that they had contact with and their level of satisfaction with these different aspects of their daily lives. We investigated relationships with family, friends and neighbours and the impact of age, health and retirement on their levels of social interaction. Each interview also incorporated a specific question on whether the interviewee was lonely, followed by a question asking them to define what the concept of 'loneliness' meant to them. This was considered important for gaining an understanding of exactly what loneliness means to older people; a dimension that has been conspicuous by its absence in previous research. Articulating older people's definition and conceptualisation of loneliness enables us to develop a more sophisticated understanding of this rather difficult to define concept.

In addition we explicitly asked participants to suggest ways in which loneliness and isolation could be ameliorated. All interviews were transcribed in full and thematic analysis was carried out using a framework constructed through 15 previously conducted pilot interviews.

Findings

Our findings are presented in three sections: response rates and the characteristics of the samples; patterns of loneliness; causes and pathways into loneliness.

Study response rate and the characteristics of the samples

The index Omnibus Survey waves included 1598 older people, of whom 1323 gave their consent to participation in our survey. At follow-up 24 of these addresses were subsequently found to be ineligible, leaving a potential study population of 1299. Of this number 243 refused (19 per cent) and 57 were not contactable (4 per cent) giving a study population of 999 respondents: response rate of 77 per cent of those eligible for the study and 63 per cent of those who participated in the index waves of the Omnibus Survey.

Our population approximates to the general population of older people living in the community in Great Britain, although our sample appears to have slightly more widows (39 per cent compared with 33 per cent) and slightly fewer women (53 per cent compared with 57 per cent). These potential biases may be important given previous research identifying increased loneliness among women and the widowed. Rates of chronic illness approximate to national norms for older people living in the community (Table 6.1), although we appear to have an under-representation of those with sight and hearing problems. Approximately one third of our sample, 37 per cent, lived alone and levels of social contact were consistent with the established national pattern.

Prevalence and patterns of loneliness

The prevalence of loneliness

The majority of participants, 61 per cent, rated themselves as 'never' lonely, 31 per cent as 'sometimes' lonely, 5 per cent as 'often' lonely

Table 6.1 Characteristics of sample

	GB 2001	ESRC 2001
Demographic		
Lives alone	37	37
Female	57	53
Age 75+	42	42
Widowed	33	39
Material resources		
Car owner	56	58
Home owner	68	72
Health		
Longstanding illness	61	62
Problems with sight	27	24
Problems with hearing	41	36
Social contact		
See family weekly	66	62
Phone family weekly	85	81
See friends weekly	70	71
Phone friends weekly	67	64
See neighbours weekly	88	89

and 2 per cent as always lonely (see Table 6.2). By inviting respondents to compare their levels of loneliness now as compared with a decade earlier we could start to investigate age-related patterns of loneliness. Approximately two-thirds (68 per cent) of our participants reported that their loneliness rating had not changed in the previous decade while 23 per cent reported that it had deteriorated. However, change was not always universally for the worse as 10 per cent of participants rated themselves as less lonely than a decade previous. Approximately half of the lonely respondents reported that they experienced this at particular times, most frequently at the weekends (Table 6.2).

In terms of preceding cohort patterns of loneliness three interrelated trends are evident (Table 6.3). First, there is a remarkable degree of consistency in the percentage of respondents rating themselves as 'always/often' lonely across the studies. For example, in 1948 Sheldon reported that 8 per cent of his sample were always/often lonely

Table 6.2 Extent of loneliness and time spent alone

	n	%
Loneliness		
Always	16	2
Often	49	5
Sometimes	320	32
Never	612	61
More lonely than 10 years ago		
More	301	23
Same	605	68
Less	90	10
Lonely at specific periods		
Yes	208	54
No	177	46
Times most often lonely		
Morning	29	14
Afternoon	21	10
Evening	138	67
Week	93	47
Weekend	58	30
Holiday periods	14	7
Other	31	16

compared with 7 per cent in our survey. However, there is an obvious change in the percentages reporting that they were sometimes or never lonely. The former category has changed from 13 per cent in 1948 to 32 per cent in 2001. Similarly the percentages rating themselves as never lonely have decreased. Examination of cohort changes in specific groups of older people is shown in Table 6.4. The prevalence of loneliness among the single and those living alone appears to have decreased while for the widowed this may have increased. However, such data should be interpreted with caution because of the small sample sizes and large confidence intervals.

The 'risk factors' for loneliness were grouped into four main domains: socio-demographic, material resources, health resources, social resources and social network. Nineteen individual variables were associated with increased reported rates of loneliness at the univariate

Table 6.3 Prevalence of loneliness in different studies

	% lonely		
	Always	**Sometimes**	**Never**
Sheldon (1948)	8	13	79
Townsend (1957)	5	22	72
Townsend (1968)	5	22	73
Tunstall (1966)	9	25	66
ESRC (2001)	7	32	61

Table 6.4 Percentage always/often lonely in different studies

Factor	Sheldon (1948)	Townsend (1968)	ESRC study (2001)
Age			
65–74	7		6
75–84	9		13
85+	13		18
Sex			
Male	7	5	8
Female	6	8	11
Marital status			
Married	–	3	1
Widowed/divorced	14	11	18
Single	13	5	9
Living alone	32	17	17

level of analysis (6.5). This pattern confirms the established one (Victor et al. 2000). However, these dimensions are clearly interrelated and a multivariate analysis was undertaken, the results of which are summarised in Table 6.5. Six major factors, independent of each other, place older people vulnerable to the risk of reporting loneliness. These are three demographic factors: marital status, with all groups vulnerable when compared with married elders, time alone and reported increases in loneliness. Then there were three health variables that appeared to be linked with vulnerability to loneliness: a high GHQ score,

Table 6.5 The correlates of loneliness

	Univariate analysis	Mulitivariate analysis
Personal circumstances		
↑ Age	✓	Protective
Female	✓	
Widowhood	✓	Vulnerability
Living alone	✓	
Material resources		
Tenure	✓	
Qualifications	✓	Protective
Car ownership	✓	
Health resources		
Hearing problems	✓	
Sight problems	✓	
Longstanding illness	✓	
Mental ill health	✓	Vulnerability
Poor health rating	✓	Vulnerability
Diagnosis of depression	✓	
Poor health expectation	✓	Vulnerability
Social resources		
Time alone	✓	Vulnerability
Increased loneliness	✓	Vulnerability
Support in crisis	✓	
Activities in last week	✓	
Days out of the house	✓	
Increase in time alone	✓	

an indirect indicator of poor mental health, poor evaluation of current health and worse than expected health in later life. Two factors appear 'protective' against loneliness – advanced age and possession of educational qualifications, although this latter factor was a borderline statistical significance.

Types of loneliness

Following the protocol outlined above we identified a fourfold typology of loneliness. Just over half of the sample (53 per cent) were defined as

119

never lonely; 15 per cent were identified as the consistently lonely group; 29 per cent of the group were classified as increasingly lonely while 10 per cent were characterised by decreased levels of loneliness.

Older people's perspectives on loneliness

One of the key aims of the qualitative study was to explore older people's experiences and understanding of loneliness and the kinds of interventions they felt would ameliorate loneliness. From our respondents we were able to distinguish three major definitions of loneliness and three distinct pathways into and through loneliness. The pathways reflect the temporal nature of the experience of loneliness that respondents saw as a feature of loneliness, which could ebb and flow across the life course. The pathways also reflect the groups derived from loneliness theory: the existentialist, characterised by 'primary loneliness', and the 'secondary' loneliness group for whom loneliness arose as a response to a change in circumstances, usually a loss of some type such as bereavement or severe illness.

Definitions of loneliness

Three distinct definitional categories emerged when respondents were asked specifically how they would define loneliness. These were social network definitions; functional or structural definitions and personality-based definitions.

The network definition was used either singly or in combination as the factor that defined loneliness for 32/44 respondents. In the eyes of our respondents loneliness is linked to the number and closeness, both spatially and qualitatively, of relationships with friends and relations. Explanations for loneliness were couched in terms of dislocated social networks, in terms of a spouse, family or friends, or some combination of these factors. Such definitions reflect a conceptualisation of loneliness as a response to changes in other aspects of an individual's life:

> Loneliness ... It can be almost physical ... I've got everything but I haven't got enough. I ... er ... you can never replace a wife. You can never replace a partner. You can't turn it on and off like a tap. If you love somebody for that many years, it's a very lonely life.

Two other definitions of loneliness were advanced more rarely. A functional definition relates to the loss of a range of abilities and structural limitations imposed upon by daily life by reduced income and access to transport, etc. Again this is a view of loneliness as a secondary response to changing circumstances. The state of mind definition of loneliness conceptualises it as being 'caused' solely by an individual's personal state of mind. This, perhaps, reflects the notion of primary loneliness where this is viewed as part of the make-up of the particular individual:

> I don't think there's any real excuse for loneliness, it might be harder for some people than others to get out, not to feel lonely, but if you make an effort it's not necessary ... It's just that there are so many things today to help people, to bring them out, to get them to mix with others. I mean there are so many things, there are so many voluntary things that you can join, you don't have to sit back bemoaning your fate and feeling lonely. I'd assume a lot of it is self-induced surely?

None of the minority of people who classified loneliness as a state of mind or a failing of personal attitude classified themselves as lonely. Therefore seeing loneliness in this way was seeing a failure in the attitude of someone else rather than a failure in yourself.

Types of loneliness

Respondents felt that there was a very strong temporal component to the experience of loneliness which could vary across the life course, over the year, across the week and across that day. Two distinct trajectories were implied: acute where the onset of loneliness resulted from an acute change in circumstances in contrast to a more insidious mode of onset (and by implication reduction of loneliness). From the responses we identified four distinct categories that mirror those used in the quantitative study. Leaving aside the 'never lonely' group, we identified the following typology.

The regenerative group identifies those who become less lonely across their life course. The exemplars of the gradualist pathway were: three never married women who reported more pressure to be social, have partners, get married, and have children when they were younger. With age they became less lonely and more able to cope with being alone, and with other people's opinions of the fact that they were alone. This category also identifies those experiences of loneliness that were usually caused by a specific traumatic event of some kind – loss of a partner or severe, restrictive health problems and who, over the course of time, adapted to the new circumstances in which they found themselves and gradually became less lonely:

> I was widowed almost two years ago and of course that was very difficult because I'd nursed my husband at home, and of course he was blind for years before that so everything did close in on us a lot. But since then ... erm ... OK, so I've joined the Townswomen's Guild, I only went on one meeting and I went on one trip to Poole. So I did go to evening classes and took an intermediate thing on word processing because I wanted to update my system. Apart from that I've done various classes and I've been helping my daughter who's a recovering alcoholic, but we don't talk about that ... I've got the dog who I walk twice a day, in this weather that's great ... I do a lot in the garden ... Basically I suppose I'm a lot better off that I was last time you interviewed me, I'm very lucky.

The increasing loneliness trajectory describes a pattern of intensifying of experiences of loneliness across the life course. Again we can differentiate between those whose experiences of loneliness emerged gradually and those where it emerged following a single, specific event, usually bereavement, or a series of events which acted as a trigger such as friends moving away or dying, changing neighbourhoods, retirement, and children moving away, which resulted, either directly or indirectly, in a reduction in the social interaction available to the person.

> You get very lonely because you can't see any purpose. It's the purpose; you need a purpose in life.

> But now we find that as you're getting older you're losing friends. Because we've lost two or three friends that have died recently, you know, and you don't make new ones. I suppose it's because we don't go out. I'm working and we don't go out socially, so you don't really meet new people.

The existential loneliness trajectory conceptualises the experience of loneliness as a constant theme and experience across the life course and was the least common of the trajectories identified. Although the intensity of loneliness varied across time, there was always an underlying awareness. One woman talked about the constant fear of being lonely and the fact that she hated being alone, no matter where, or what time of day or night, or for how long. This is clearly an extreme example of existential loneliness, where being lonely, and the fear of being lonely, completely takes over the life of the respondent.

Causes and prevention of loneliness

Respondents were asked explicitly what they thought were the causes of loneliness and what could be done to ameliorate the problem. Twenty-seven individual factors grouped into four major domains were identified as 'causes' of loneliness. Again family and friendship networks were seen as the major influencing factor as to whether an older person would experience loneliness. Community networks, activities and functional limitations were also cited as important predisposing factors. Less importance was attributed to 'personality' factors.

Discussion and conclusion

Loneliness is still conceptualised by many, including older people themselves, as a problem which is specific to old age, despite the evidence that other groups within the population are also likely to experience this state (Ellaway et al. 1999). Major British community studies have reported rates of loneliness in people over the age of 65 ranging from 5 per cent to 16 per cent (Sheldon 1948; Townsend 1957, 1968; Tunstall 1966; Hunt 1978; Bond and Carstairs 1982; Qureshi and Walker 1989) with a median of approximately 9 to 10 per cent (Victor et al. 2000). Our data is consistent with previous research in that 7 per cent reported that they were often/always lonely. However, in comparison with previous research, our participants were more likely to report that they were sometimes lonely. Almost a third of participants were in this group, which is much greater than the 11 to 22 per cent reported in previous research (Sheldon 1948; Townsend 1957). We used a direct self-report measure of loneliness that is well established but not without limitations that measures the emotional dimension of loneliness.

Clearly some groups of elders were more likely to report that they were lonely than others. Our univariate analysis identified strong relationships between loneliness and a wide range of factors that were consistent with previous research. However, many of these factors are clearly interrelated and a more complex statistical analysis revealed that there were vulnerability factors (marital status, time alone, health rating, health expectation, mental health and perceived increased loneliness) and two 'protective' factors (age and educational qualifications) (Brown and Harris 1978). These results are novel for two reasons. First, in a nationally representative sample they suggest that many of the factors commonly thought to be associated with loneliness such as gender, household status and chronic illness/disability do not demonstrate an independent relationship once the influence of confounding factors is taken into account (for example, gender is clearly linked to living alone, chronic health and widowhood).

The second novel finding relates to notions of 'protective' factors that are associated with reduced vulnerability to loneliness. Previous studies have concentrated upon identifying risk factors and have not reported results indicating attributes that are associated with less vulnerability to loneliness in later life, while this study suggested that two factors – advanced age and educational qualifications – were significantly and independently associated with lower susceptibility to loneliness. Both univariate and multivariate models such as that by Fees et al. (1999) and Wenger et al. (1996) have suggested that increased age is a risk factor for loneliness. Our study demonstrates the opposite finding. Given that it is well established that those aged 85 years and over are less likely to participate in research, this finding may be an artefact as a result of non-response bias. However, some limited support for this novel conclusion is given by the work of Holmen and Furukawa (2002). They report that among participants in a Swedish ten-year follow-up of those aged 75+ rates of loneliness fell from 35.6 per cent (always/often/sometimes lonely) to 4.6 per cent at the third follow-up. This suggests the influence of two interrelated factors: a survivor effect where those who are lonely exhibit elevated mortality/ morbidity and do not survive to advanced ages in the community (either dying or being admitted to long-stay care); an adaptive response where those who do survive 'adapt' to the vicissitudes of old age such as bereavement or declining health. This links with our 'vulnerability' factors that relate, in large measure, to the expectations of older people and to our trajectories of loneliness where some study participants report decreasing levels of loneliness. Clearly this is an area for further research.

One characteristic of existing research in this field is that it presupposes a common understanding of what it is to be lonely and has rarely examined older people's understanding of loneliness and what they are trying to convey when they describe themselves in this way. This links to the fact that the majority of studies carried out have been quantitative rather than qualitative in nature (O'Connor 1994; Russell and Schofield 1999) and highly untheoretical in approach. Hence, as well as trying to examine trends over time and current patterns, there is a need to examine older people's understandings of the key issue of loneliness and to develop our theoretical and conceptual under-standing of these aspects of later life. Older people in this study identified loneliness as predominantly a secondary response to either acute or chronic changes in circumstances. Predominantly loneliness was conceptualised in terms of deficits in the quality and quantity of the social networks of individuals. This seems to be more in line with the 'social' rather than emotional definition of loneliness.

We developed a novel typology of loneliness. This distinguished between those who had always been lonely, those for whom old age was characterised by increased feelings of loneliness, and those for whom the opposite was true. This type of approach generates varying esti-mates of the extent of loneliness in later life. The majority of respondents were defined as never lonely, while 15 per cent were the existentialist or consistently lonely group. For 10 per cent loneliness levels had decreased, and for 20 per cent they had increased. This highlights the 'dynamic' nature of the concepts of isolation and loneliness and indicates that 'single point in time' prevalence rates may be of limited utility and that single policy solutions may not be appropriate (Wenger and Burholt 2003).

Respondents defined loneliness as deriving from three sets of factors: impaired social networks, 'functional/environmental' impairments and 'personality' factors. As such these influenced the kinds of interven-tions they felt could combat loneliness and isolation, which included enhancing social networks, promoting a sense of neighbourliness/ community, developing a portfolio of 'appropriate' activities and attending to structural barriers to participation including transport and financial provision for later life.

Loneliness clearly compromises the quality of life of the older per-son. Hence we need to design and implement interventions that are appropriate to the needs of this population. Our evidence suggests that loneliness in later life is not a single homogeneous experience and there are different 'pathways' into loneliness in later life. Different factors may underline such trajectories and this needs to be recognised in designing appropriate interventions which also respond to the needs of different groups of elders.

Acknowledgements

We are very pleased to acknowledge the bodies that funded this research, our collaborators and the Office of National Statistics who conducted the fieldwork. The research was funded by the Economic and Social Research Council (award number L480254042) as part of the Growing Older Programme. The Quality of Life Survey was also part funded by grants held by Professor Ann Bowling (grant L480254043 – also part of the Growing Older programme) and Professor Shah Ebrahim (Medical Research Council Health Services Research Collaboration). We are grateful to the Office for National Statistics (ONS) Omnibus Survey Unit for overseeing the fieldwork and preparing the data set. Those who carried out the original analysis and collection of the data hold no responsibility for the further analysis and interpretation of them. Material from the ONS Omnibus Survey, made available through ONS, has been used with the permission of the Controller of The Stationery Office. The dataset will be held at the ESRC Data Archive at Essex University. Finally, we would like to thank the ONS interviewers and we are also indebted to all those older people who gave so freely of their time to participate in this study.

7

Older men – their health behaviours and partnership status

Kate Davidson and Sara Arber

Introduction

Only comparatively recently has there been sociological interest in the health behaviours of older men and a recognition that the health and well-being of men cannot be separated from their socially constructed roles. For too long the medical model, focusing on pathological aspects of causality, has dominated health research on older men. Much attention has been paid, for example, to the effects of smoking, drinking, poor diet and lack of exercise on morbidity rates as the principal causes of older male mortality: coronary heart disease, stroke and cancer. Less attention has been paid to the meanings of health risk to older men and how these intersect with class, partnership status and notions of appropriate masculine behaviour.

Researching older men

There is comparatively little sociological study on men after retirement age and Thompson (1994: 1–21) has offered four principal reasons for this relative invisibility. First, not only are there fewer men in the older population, but just under three-quarters of these are married and living in their own home with a spouse (ONS 2002a). Men do suffer a mortality disadvantage, but they tend to experience more 'catastrophic' illness, dying sooner than women who are more likely to suffer long-standing chronic debilitating illness (Kalache 2002). Second, owing to more stable employment histories and higher earnings, older men are more likely than women to be in receipt of occupational or private pensions as well as a full state pension. Although their income is considerably less than that of mid-life men, it is higher than that of older women (Ginn 2003). Policy research addresses problem-orientated issues that have focused on the relative disadvantage for older women: their longevity, poverty, disability and social care needs. Thus, older men are rendered less visible to health and social services. Third, in academia, 'gender studies' have come to be synonymous with 'women's studies'. Clearly, 'gender' means both men and women, yet recognition of this was somewhat lost in the feminist discourse of the late twentieth century. Fourth, the study of 'masculinity' has also ignored older men in its focus on the meaning of manhood and its impact on, for example, sporting activity, crime, violence and sexuality (Kimmel and Messner 2001). Little research has been carried out on the different experiences of older men compared to younger men and of older men compared to older women of the same generation (Thompson 1994).

The main focus of this chapter is to examine older men's attitudes to health maintenance in terms of subjective individual health behaviours (primary prevention), and to objective health protective strategies in terms of the use of health professional advice and health screening (secondary prevention). It explores the extent to which primary and secondary prevention of ill health relates to partnership status and living arrangements of men over the age of 65 years. Marital status is an important determinant of health behaviour for men, with married men advantaged since there is substantial evidence that women have a primary role in maintaining a family 'health watch' which may be increasingly salient in later life (Davidson and Arber 2003). There are implications for the quality of life experienced by older men depending upon partnership status and its influence on primary and secondary health protection activities. For example, the singer Johnny Cash, who died aged 71 in September 2003 a bare four months after the death of his second wife, June Carter Cash, maintained that she was the greatest influence on his health behaviours and quality of life and credited her with turning his life around from alcohol and drug abuse, and supporting him during their 35-year marriage:

What June did for me was post signs along the way, lift me when I was weak, encourage me when I was discouraged, and love me when I was alone and felt unlovable. She is the greatest woman I have ever known. Nobody else, except my mother, comes close.

(johnnycash.com 2003)

Older men, partnership status and quality of life

Partnership status in the ageing population is projected to undergo considerable change over the next two decades. The 2001 UK Census data show that over the age of 65, 72 per cent of men compared to 39 per cent of women live with their spouse (StatBase 2002). However, demographic trends suggest that an increasing proportion of men over the age of 65 will live alone in their later years: almost one in four at present which is projected to rise to one in three over the next generation (Davies et al. 1998). Among men currently aged 65 and over living in the community, 17 per cent are widowed, while only 7 per cent are never married and 5 per cent are divorced or separated (StatBase 2002). By 2021, however, it is projected that the proportion of divorced men over 65 will increase rapidly to 13 per cent while the proportion who are widowed will fall to 13 per cent, mainly because of improvements in mortality, and 8 per cent will be never married (Government Actuary's Department 2001).

Older men who live without women are more likely to lack the health protective support experienced by partnered men. They are also more likely to have reduced informal social networks since these too are most frequently generated and maintained by women throughout the life course (Scott and Wenger 1995: 58–172). Research has also found that older men without partners are more likely to live in residential care, despite having lower average levels of disability than lone older women (Arber and Ginn 1995; Tinker 1997). Therefore, we argue that there are implications not only for policy-making decisions on a macro level, but for the quality of life of lone older men in the twenty-first century.

Quality of life as defined by the World Health Organisation is a complex concept which incorporates, among other issues, health and social well-being:

an individual's perception of his or her position in life in the context of the culture and value system where they live, and in relation to their goals and expectations, standards and concerns. It is a broad ranging concept, incorporating in a complex way, a person's physical health, psychological state, level of independence, social relationships, personal beliefs and relationships to salient features in the environment.

(WHO 2002: 13)

Recent UK policy initiatives have been a response to growing awareness of the importance of health maintenance in later life on individual, institutional and societal levels. The National Service Framework for Older People set eight 'standards' for the care of older people across health and social services. Standard Eight is *The promotion of health and active life in older age*. The rationale states:

There is a growing body of evidence to suggest that the modification of risk factors for disease even late in life can have health benefits for the individual; longer life, increased or maintained levels of functional ability, disease prevention and an improved sense of well-being. Integrated strategies for older people aimed at promoting good health and quality of life, and to prevent or delay frailty and disability can have significant benefits for the individual and society.

(DoH 2001: 107)

It is well documented that within the ageing male population there are distinct worldwide regional and cultural differences in morbidity and mortality rates (Kinsella 1997). In the UK alone, a man with a history of working in a professional occupation and living in South-East England, is likely to outlive his unskilled manual compatriot in Scotland by some 11 years, with a projected life expectancy of 83 years compared to 71 years (StatBase 2002). Work history and work conditions, and for this cohort of older men experience of armed conflict, will also influence long-term health. Occupational accidents now cause less morbidity and mortality in men in the UK but were prevalent in the earlier years of this older generation.

Older men and health behaviour

Figure 7.1 is a model that explores the determinants for men's health in later life. Two important elements in health status are biological and social factors which in turn are contingent on two 'lynchpin' determinants contextualised within economic and cultural circumstances.

The biologically gendered experience of morbidity and mortality in

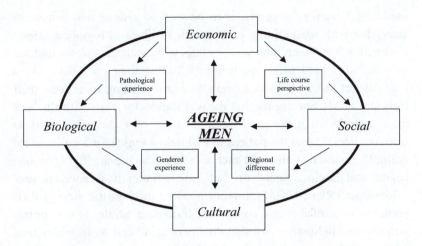

Figure 7.1 Determinants of older men's health in later life

later life is well documented in the medical literature (Kalache 2000). However, it is essential to examine economic, social and cultural differences and to what extent regional variations, local, national and global, impact on health behaviours. Figure 7.1 shows simplified pathways to the understanding of older men's health. Access to economic resources has a bearing on health and life expectancy. Health and wealth are directly correlated for men, but not for women (Arber and Cooper 1999). Within the life course perspective, partnership status provides an important indicator of older men's health behaviours, particularly in later life. Older married men are more likely than lone older men to have a 'caretaker' to monitor their health behaviours, or a 'gatekeeper' to encourage health consultation (Davidson and Arber 2003).

The health of men is strongly influenced by events throughout the life course and by the social construction of appropriate masculine behaviour in all societies (Kalache 2000). From an early age, females are more orientated towards treatment-seeking behaviour for a variety of conditions, whereas males learn to ignore pain and shun doctors (Hearn 1998: 12–36). Courtney (2000) argues that men take more health risks, including interpersonal violence, than women throughout their lives, and that this is primarily driven by the 'machismo imperative' to compete and to be seen to be as 'strong'. A sign of weakness, Courtney suggests, is to be seen to reduce risk behaviour associated with masculinity, or to admit to illness. Moynihan (1998) observed in her research on young males with testicular cancer that the men found it hard to accept being ill. Taking their condition 'like a man' meant hiding behind a brave face and refusing to express their fears and needs. She argues that the way the doctor deals with the 'sick man' and the language used in explanation of a condition (and its consequences) allows the patient to maintain a sense of masculinity; for example, male clinicians used such metaphors as 'a plane flying on one engine and landing safely' or that 'one cylinder is as good as two' (Moynihan 1998: 1074). Men tend to take a mechanistic view of their bodies as controllable and controlled. Indeed, as Seidler (1994) points out, this highlights the Cartesian duality of mind and body, where men separate their physical and emotional existences.

In recognition of men's greater tendency to think of their bodies as engines, the Men's Health Forum and a leading pharmaceutical company, in collaboration with the legendary Haynes car manuals, produced a step-by-step guide to men's health (Banks 2002) using the vocabulary of car mechanics. Interspersed with facts, figures and guidance on health maintenance is a cartoon character called Dipstick who translates advice into 'mechanic speak'. For example, on smoking it says: 'Cars with smoking exhausts don't look or smell healthy, and they invariably fail their MOTs' (Banks 2002: 2.7) and 'Don't end up an insurance write-off. Give up the cigs' (3.9). On alcohol consumption: 'Too many soakings will cause your filters to block and corrode. Try to drink in moderation' (6.4). In terms of health maintenance in later life it advises: 'Ageing is one thing that comes to us all, although a regular body service will help keep you running like a Rolls Royce' (2.1). The format of the manual responds to but also reinforces the mechanistic way in which many men think about their bodies. A theme that runs through the manual, however, is the encouragement to seek professional advice, to consult 'an expert', much as they would do if their car was not 'firing on all cylinders'.

It is important to recognise that the customary approach to health improvement has been to target individuals, but less attention has been paid to addressing the broad determinants of older men's health behaviours. These include biological, social, cultural and economic factors in influencing men's health protective strategies. Such a holistic approach refers not just to the biological differences between men and women, but also to the socially constructed roles that shape masculinity and femininity throughout the life course, compounded by economic and cultural influences.

Kalache (2002) suggests a need to revisit the WHO European Panel for Gender and ask further questions about the lesser use of health services by men. He argues that we need to understand men's health perceptions of their own health needs and why they may not believe that health services are appropriate for addressing them. It is the last two areas of research identified by Kalache, male risk-taking behaviours and gender differences in treatment-seeking behaviours, that are addressed in this chapter.

Methods

Using a combination of quantitative and qualitative methods, both older men's subjective awareness and objective action for health maintenance are explored. First, we analysed five years (1993–1996, 1998) of the General Household Survey (GHS), a national probability based cross-sectional survey which is conducted annually except in 1997 (OPCS 1996, 1997, 1998, 2000). Questions about self-reported physical health were asked in all the years (men 55+, n = 12342). Questions about alcohol consumption and smoking were asked in alternate years. Therefore the analysis included data from 1994, 1996 and 1998 (men 55+, n = 7179). Second, we interviewed 85 men over the age of 65 who were married/cohabiting (30), widowed (33), divorced/separated (10) and never married (12). The widowed, divorced/separated and never married men are over-represented in our sample in order to examine the lived experience of lone older men compared to those who are partnered.

The qualitative sample of older men was selected by several methods. Posters and flyers were placed in local general practitioners' (GP, family physician) surgeries and a range of different organisations which have older people in their membership, and included voluntary and statutory day centres, church, sports and leisure clubs, social clubs such as the Lions, Rotary Club, Freemasons and Royal British Legion (military veterans' organisation). However, very few respondents volunteered through this method. Following local ethical committee approval we contacted two large local GP group practices. Letters were sent out to a representative sample of men aged 65 and over on their practice lists that outlined the study and asked them to return a short questionnaire noting their marital status and previous occupation. The vast majority of respondents were married, but from the responses we were able to identify divorced, never married and widowed men for interview.

A few of the partnership histories of the older men we interviewed were complex. For example, some men had been married more than once, some had been divorced and then widowed, and some had been widowed or divorced and were now cohabiting. For the analysis, we categorised men by their current partnership status. Table 7.1 shows the partnership status and average age of each group. The divorced men were the youngest group with an average age of 68, and there were none over the age of 80. This contrasts with the oldest group, the widowers, whose average age was 79: 14 out of 33 were 80 plus, with none under 70. The average age of the 85 participants was 75.

Almost all the interviews were carried out in the home of the respondent (two were carried out in private, in a private room at the university) and the vast majority with the respondent alone. However, the wives of three of the married men wished to stay during the interview and contributed to the exchange, particularly in aiding their husband's memory or expanding an account or recollection. This raised some methodological issues of validity and reliability with

Table 7.1 Partnership status and average age of the sample of men

Partnership status	Average age
Married/cohabiting (n = 30)	73
Widowed (n = 33)	79
Divorced/separated (n = 10)	68
Never married (n = 12)	73
Total n = 85	75

potential sources of error and bias – given that the other men interviewed had no prompting. We overcame this by using the initial
responses of the men in our thematic analysis rather than those altered
following their spouse's intervention.

The interviews were taperecorded with the permission of the men
and took between 45 and 90 minutes. Confidentiality and anonymity
were guaranteed and the men were reassured that if they wished to
have the tape turned off or terminate the interview at any time they
could do so. None terminated the interview but two men, one
widowed and one divorced, requested the tape to be interrupted for a
short period while they grappled with emotional memories. The
interviews were fully transcribed and entered into a qualitative software
program, QSR NVivo, for thematic and iterative analysis (Boyatzis
1998).

Almost all the 85 interviews were carried out by a male researcher
who was over the age of 60 and the remainder by the first author. This
raised interesting issues of interviewer effect. For several decades there
has been discourse from feminist and ethnic minority research methodology on gender and race in the interview dynamic (Oakley 1975;
Bryan et al. 1985; Mason 1996). However, relatively little attention has
been paid to the effect of gender and age differences/similarities in
interviewing older people. Bury and Holme in their study of people
over the age of 90 stress that:

> In a study of this kind the interviewer is all-important. Patience and
> sympathy are essential qualities and we were fortunate in having these in
> good measure among the 12 women and 1 man who made up the team.
>
> (Bury and Holme 1990: 137)

No comment was made on the effect of a male researcher/inter-
viewer on the data, nor was there any indication of the age of the male
involved. Lee (1993: 100) quotes a survey carried out by Johnson and
Delamater in 1976 wherein male interviewers received different
reported levels of sexual behaviour by respondents, but Lee does not
indicate the age of the interviewers and how this differed from the
interviewees. In our study, we were unable to undertake comparative
analysis of interviewer effect because only four interviews were carried
out by a female researcher.

Davidson listened to the tapes in this Growing Older (GO) study, and made comparisons with her previous research on older widowed men (Davidson 1999). She found that the men in her study talked freely about their late wife, their family, previous work and social relationships and their health status. The men in the GO project, interviewed by the older male researcher, talked about their social relationships but were much more likely to talk at length about their previous occupation(s) and work history. The 'matching' of age and gender probably meant a greater rapport in an area of shared experience, that is the world of male employment. Also, the men tended to recite life successes, boastful of their achievements, but tended to be wistful for a 'lost world'. Nevertheless, in the GO project, a great deal of empathy was perceived between the researcher and his interviewees, demonstrated by their willingness to disclose sexual intimacies and detailed physical limitations, for example, their experience of impotence. Davidson found that some of her respondents talked about sex, in terms of missing intimacy with their late wife, and at times were jokingly flirtatious, but did not discuss sexual dysfunction. Therefore, although in both studies the men talked about social relationships, past employment and sexual matters, the content and emphasis differed depending upon the sex and age of the interviewer. Given the paucity of literature on age and gender effects on interviewing older people, we consider further investigation would be justified.

The theoretical orientation of the analysis was grounded in symbolic interactionism, utilising role and exchange theories and the methodology reflects this approach. Qualitative methods provide the most suitable means of access to the meanings that people assign to particular activities and experiences (Silverman 1993). The analysis was performed with the aim to develop theory 'grounded' in the data, rather than testing preconceived hypotheses. This allowed the subjective accounts of the participants to be paramount and recognised the importance of the context in which the interview was produced (Flick 2002). The software program permitted flexible coding and analytical memos from the vast amount of interview data. Foremost it allowed the use of a modified version of the 'grounded' approach of Glaser and Strauss's method of 'constant comparative analysis' (1967).

The majority of respondents were accessed through the two GP group practice lists and while we make no claim for generalisability we interviewed men from a wide range of ages and socio-economic groups.

However, it must be recognised that the men were self-selected as they responded to our letter and agreed to being interviewed in their home. We are mindful of the small numbers of divorced and never married men and we make no claims for generalisability.

Findings: the quantitative data

Older men's self reported health

Our analysis of the GHS data sets revealed that lone men were more likely to report poor health than partnered men (Figure 7.2). Divorced men consistently report the poorest health across the three age groups: 55 to 64, 65 to 74 and 75 and over. Widowed men between the ages of 55 and 64 reported poorer health than older groups of widowers. This may be an effect of the unexpectedness of widowhood for men in this age group, which causes them to experience a much reduced quality of life and consequential poor health. The reduced percentage of those reporting poor health among single men over 75 may reflect that it is

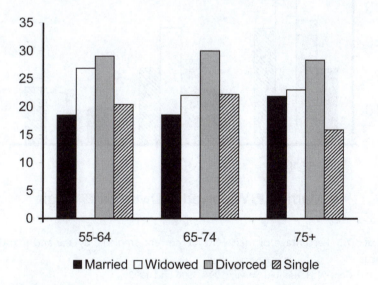

Figure 7.2 Percentage of older men who report poor health by age and marital status
Source: General Household Survey 1993, 1994, 1995, 1996 and 1998
(see base numbers in Appendix, Table A7.1)
Authors' analysis

principally those who are in reasonable or good health who can still live in the community. Married men report the best health in each age group except for those aged 75 and over.

Health risk behaviours

In 1994, 1996 and 1998 the GHS asked questions about smoking and alcohol consumption. Figure 7.3 shows current smokers by age and marital status. Divorced older men in each age group were the most likely to smoke, except from above 75 when divorced and never married older men were equally likely to smoke. Married older men are least likely to be smokers in each age group, apart from over 75, when widowed and married men have an equally low prevalence of smoking. Widowers aged 55 to 64 have a high level of smoking, 35 per cent, almost as high as for divorced men in this age group, but the relatively high levels of smoking among widowers decreases with advancing age.

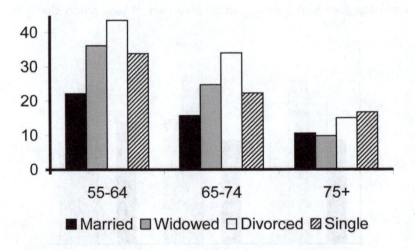

Figure 7.3 Percentage of men who are current smokers, by age and marital status
Source: General Household Survey 1994, 1996 and 1998
(See base numbers in Appendix, Table A7.2)
Authors' analysis

Figure 7.4 shows consumption of alcohol over the recommended weekly limit of 21 units by age and marital status. One unit of alcohol

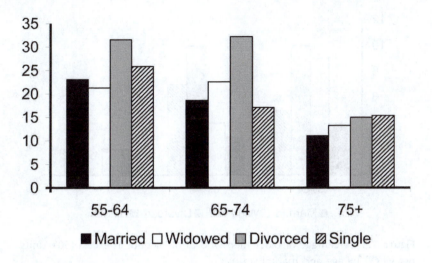

Figure 7.4 Percentage of men who consume alcohol above 21 units per week by age and marital status
Source: General Household Survey 1994, 1996 and 1998
(See base numbers in Appendix, Table A7.2)
Authors' analysis

is equivalent to a glass of wine, half a pint of beer or one measure of spirits.

Alcohol consumption decreases with age, but approximately 30 per cent of divorced men consistently report drinking over the recommended weekly limit of 21 units. Married men, however, also report consumption over the 'safe' limit, at approximately 20 per cent. Alcohol consumption in excess of 50 units per week is also more likely to be reported by divorced men aged 55 to 74 at 10 per cent (except those over 75, when it is low for all marital groups) (see Figure 7.5). Nine per cent of widowers between 55 and 64 also report drinking to excess, but this rate is halved after the age of 65. Once again, the unexpectedness of widowhood in the younger age group of men may effect a temporary increase in alcohol consumption.

Therefore, a picture emerges of older married men who report better health and fewer health damaging behaviours than men who live alone. The divorced older men reported the poorest health and greatest prevalence of health risk behaviours, while the widowers varied by age: the younger the widower, the more likely he was to report poor health

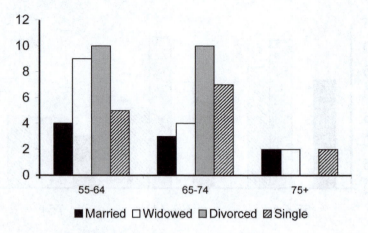

Figure 7.5 Percentage of older men who drink alcohol in excess (50+ units per week) by age and marital status
Source: General Household Survey 1994, 1996 and 1998
(See base numbers in Appendix, Table A7.2)
Authors' analysis

and risky health behaviours. The qualitative component of our research sought to answer questions as to how older men themselves viewed their health and health maintenance strategies.

The qualitative interviews with older men

What emerged from the qualitative analysis was a complex picture of health awareness, protection strategies and risk taking. Interestingly, most men knew what they 'should' do to maintain health and good quality of life, both subjectively, in reducing life-threatening practices, and objectively, in undertaking regular health screening such as monitoring blood pressure and cholesterol levels. We could surmise that older men are aware of health promotion information but, similar to other groups in society, they do not always adhere to advice.

Jon (72, married): I should walk more. I suppose if I walk round to the postbox round the corner, that's the furthest I go during the week. We try and walk at weekends. ... I'm a bad lad I know. Like for breakfast, I will get up in the morning and probably have two pots of tea, bad for you, eight cups of tea, eight spoonfuls of sugar – wrong. It used to be 16, but I have cut the sugar down. Lunch I might have a cheese sandwich, bad for me again. But then I have an evening meal. It would be a cooked meal. Last night it was bacon, tonight it will be a small roast. I like a drink, I probably drink too much, more than what I should do.

Jon was certainly not unusual in knowing what was 'bad' for him. However, for the population of older men, the results of ignoring such advice can be more catastrophic than for younger generations, given that men continue to be at higher risk than women of life-threatening ill health in later life.

This is not to say that men do not heed health advice, but in our sample only four men attended well man clinics and blood pressure and cholesterol screening sessions (as opposed to diagnostic procedures) and they were all married and tended to be under the age of 75:

Richard (69, married): Well, if there's anything going free to do with health, I usually try to get onto it. I did do a men's health course through Age Concern, a ten-week course about 18 months ago. And if I go to an exhibition somewhere or to an air show, something like that, and they do a blood test and blood pressure, I'll go in and do it, because it's there.

More commonly, lone men said they knew there were opportunities for a 'check-up', but they did not take them up.

Reg (70, divorced): Actually, I've been offered one. I suppose I ought to, really.

He went on to say that he only goes 'as and when' and this seems too often.

Common to each partnership status were men who said they seldom consulted their GP. These non-attending men could be categorised into those who were 'sceptics' and 'stoics'. The sceptics used phrases like 'most of them are a waste of time'. Clive (72, married) said: 'I don't like doctors, I keep as far away from the place ... it's not an exact science – you can quote me on that.' He went on to say that medicine was about as accurate as weather forecasting in the UK. Kevin (75, widowed) said that he would rather go to a veterinary surgeon than a doctor 'after the way they treated my wife'. Even if he had cancer, he said, he would put up with it, rather than seek medical help. The 'stoics' accepted, without complaint conditions which might, for others, prompt medical consultation, and said things like:

Paul (67, divorced): I don't give in. Even if I felt awful, I wouldn't tell anyone.

Richard (70, never married): I've always tended to think, well, it's going to go away.

Edward (71, never married): You've just got to get through it.

Most of these 'non-attenders' reported good general health, some attributed it to heredity and luck, and others to 'looking after themselves':

Andrew (75, married): I am healthy, yes. No, I've never been ill in my life. I always say I don't hold with illness. You know, it's a thing for other people. I think my good health is hereditary.

Rory (84, married): I'm one of these lucky people that have suffered good health all my life. ... we are sensible about our eating, we try and do a certain amount of walking exercise each day.

However, there was a surprisingly high reportage of asthma for which the men were prescribed an inhaler after diagnosis. In the UK it is possible to request a repeat prescription from a surgery without having to see the GP and while indeed these men were *not* visiting a doctor, they were still officially undergoing treatment. Jon (72, married) said, 'I am asthmatic I try not to suffer from it ... and being an asthmatic what I try to do is, although I do have it, I try not to suffer.' Interestingly, Jon, who believed that what 'comes by itself goes by itself', took regular medication for his asthma, but did not view this as 'treatment' because he felt in control of the asthma, by refusing to let himself 'suffer' with it.

There were a number of men who had undergone major treatment/ surgery for heart disease (usually a by-pass) or cancer (most commonly prostate) and who saw their physician for regular check-ups – from quarterly to biennially. 'They tell you to come back, you have to see them once a year, and he sort of puts the old stethoscope on, asks a few questions and tells you to come back next year' (Jeremy, 68, married). The men who reported these visits did not see them as 'sickness' consultations and tended not count them as 'going to the doctor' until the interviewer probed, often later in the interview. That is, the men said they rarely went to a doctor when originally asked, and then later disclosed a longer term condition which required regular follow-up health visits and/or repeat prescriptions for medication. These men were similar to the 'stoics', visiting their doctors only on a 'routine compliance' basis because they were requested to attend, rather than having instigated the consultation themselves.

Poor health and older men

About a fifth of the men were very ill and in need of considerable health professional input. In this group the most frequent account was of what we have termed 'domino pathology', whereby the men said they were 'perfectly healthy' until 'x' years before (commonly two to five), and then 'everything started to go wrong'. Interestingly, these stories were most often told by widowers who had cared long term for an ailing wife and could date their health decline from the death of their spouse.

> *Forrest (widowed)*: I'm now 81 and I'm in poor health, very poor health. Up until the age of 75, I was going fine and then I had a serious cancer operation. After that, everything seemed to break down.

Forrest's wife had died six years previously, after a long-term illness which required 24-hour care and he was diagnosed with cancer of the prostate three months after her death. This was not an uncommon account across the widowers. It was as though they were unable to give themselves permission to be ill while they were caring, but when this responsibility was removed ill health tumbled in. The widowers were very concerned about the prospect of deteriorating health and to what extent they would get support, or importantly become a 'burden' to an adult child, or if one was not available, other more distant family members (commonly, a niece).

The fear of becoming a burden was more likely to be explicitly expressed by the older widowers than the older divorced and never married men. Divorced and never married men were also concerned about deteriorating health, but were less likely to mention the possibility of being cared for by an adult relative either because none was available, or they did not have the sort of relationship they could fall back on when the need arose. For the never married men in particular there was an underlying assumption that if they were very ill one day they might 'have to go into a home', which reflects a long-term understanding that they were without a close family network in their later years.

The group of widowers was on average older than the other men in the sample, and were more likely to report poor health than the married men. Despite the difference in age profile, the divorced men who were younger were just as likely to report comparable serious health problems to the older widowers, but the widowers were more likely to have seen a doctor recently, that is within the previous three months. Divorced men, however, were more likely to report stress as a cause of ill health, and considered that it was a condition they had to sort out for themselves. 'The answer is, if you can't deal with it yourself, you ought to be able to' (Paul, 67).

When Dan, 72, went for help for what he thought was stress during an acrimonious divorce, he reported that his GP said, 'Oh, it is a little bit of depression you have got, but not bad enough to put you on tablets. I'm not giving you tablets because you are strong enough to weather it out.' Moynihan (1998) reported that the attitude of doctors to men can reinforce the notion of masculine 'strength of character' in coping with mental health problems. Dan was pleased in the end that he did not have medication, but commented that there was not much point in visiting the GP if he took no notice (as Dan saw it) of his mental and physical needs.

Married men also reported some very dramatic health problems, but were much more likely to say they were contented with their life despite their poor health status. The married men were also very likely to talk about their prevailing ailment(s) at some length, giving graphic details of the history, diagnosis and treatment of their condition. These men generally said they were 'lucky' to have such good family support and did not mention being or becoming a burden. There was a tacit understanding, supported by each wife, that she was happy to look after him 'in sickness and in health' (Davidson et al. 2000), a possibility no longer available to widowers or indeed divorced men.

In contrast, the never married older men talked very little about their health, despite the presence of prostate and heart problems, other than to say it was generally good, and were mostly contented with their life. These men demonstrated a stoicism which was voiced in terms of 'I'm pretty good for my age'. Their expectation was that they would need to 'deal' with ill health and would 'just have to get on with life'.

As discussed above, it is probable that when never married men reach the point where they need support, they would be more likely to enter institutional care. We interviewed never married men while they were still in the community, and as such were a relatively healthy group of respondents.

Health risk behaviours

Smoking

Only a few of the 85 men currently smoked but most were ex-smokers. For those who had given up when younger, the principal reason for cessation was financial: for example, 'Once we had the children and the mortgage, we couldn't afford to smoke' (Percy, 81, married). Deterioration in health in either self or partner was the reason offered for those who ceased smoking in later life. Those few who continued to smoke reported poor health and difficulty with walking very far. This group all volunteered that it is unwise to continue smoking, but found they could not quit.

It was deemed important by all the men that they remained physically active for as long as possible, and most continued to walk several miles a week. Some, principally married and widowed men, belonged to sports and leisure clubs, including golf, bowls, ramblers, swimming and dancing clubs. Those unable to cover any great distance or partake in a wide range of physical activities emphasised how far they could actually manage and how much they could do.

Alcohol consumption

There were differences in alcohol consumption patterns between the partnership categories. The married men were more likely to report their alcohol intake as regular but moderate. This finding is supported by Ward (1997) who also reported that older married women are more likely than partnerless women to consume a regular but moderate amount of alcohol. This reflects the more companionate drinking habits of couples and their friends. The widowers reported the least alcohol consumption, although some said they had 'hit the bottle' for a while in early bereavement, which is supported in the quantitative analysis (Figure 7.5). The divorced and never married men were the more likely to report two extremes: total abstinence or excessive intake.

In both these latter categories, there were abstainers who said they were recovering alcoholics (see also Appendix to chapter).

Discussion and conclusion

Although mediated by gender, ethnicity, class and geographical location, failing health is a virtual certainty at some point in old age. There was a disjuncture between what the older men knew about subjective and objective health maintenance strategies, and how they ultimately acted on this knowledge. We argue that notions of independence and masculinity in health matters identified in younger generations of men (Courtney 2000) persist into late life and continue to influence decisions on seeking professional health care. However, partnered men were more likely to seek help and take appropriate advice following consultation than men who lived alone.

For men who have had little or no 'ongoing contact' with health professionals (unlike most women) in their life course, it seems unlikely that they will turn to the health sector when they reach later life. Whilst most women have routinely visited the doctor through the life course, for family planning, pregnancy, or to take their children for clinics' immunisation programmes as well as when they are sick, the men in this study seemed to consider going to the doctor as a sign of weakness. They did not want to be seen to 'give in' to sickness. However, doctor avoidance becomes a vicious circle. The men interviewed admitted to postponing making an appointment until they were very sick. They then have negative associations with the doctor, whom they see when they are in pain or feel very unwell and, importantly, who may give them bad news about their health.

There are many serious conditions that are 'symptom free', that is the person does not necessarily know they are suffering because they cannot identify an effect such as pain. These conditions include high blood pressure, Type II diabetes, cardiac abnormalities, some cancers and early liver and kidney failure. However, once they attend a doctor for one complaint such as breathlessness (the first domino), examination and further tests might reveal underlying long-standing chronic disease with multiple health consequences.

To date, most health education has been directed at individuals and has been based on a limited understanding of their social condition.

In order to generate substantial and effective changes in the health-related behaviours of older men, interventions need to be sensitive to the economic, biological, social and cultural constructs that shape the expectations and behaviour of men as they age and experience health transitions.

Acknowledgements

We are grateful to the National Statistics for permission to use the General Household Survey data and to the UK Data Archive and Manchester Computing Centre for access to the data. This research was funded by the Economic and Social Research Council.

Appendix

Table A7.1 Base numbers of men by age group for Figure 7.2 – self-assessed health

	55–64	65–74	75+	55+
Married	4238	3533	1655	9426
Widowed	186	508	799	1493
Divorced	358	230	67	655
Never married	348	288	132	768
Total	5130	4559	2653	12342

Source: *General Household Survey*, 1993, 1994, 1995, 1996 and 1998 (authors' analysis)

Table A7.2 Base numbers of men by age group for figures 7.3, 7.4, 7.5

	55–64	65–74	75+	55+
Married	2428	1992	1007	5427
Widowed	108	315	491	914
Divorced	209	153	34	396
Never married	201	175	66	442
Total	2946	2635	1598	7179

Source: *General Household Survey*, 1994, 1996 and 1998 (authors' analysis)

8

A participatory approach to older women's quality of life

Joanne Cook, Tony Maltby and Lorna Warren

Introduction

This chapter reports an innovative, qualitative project which sought to adopt a methodological approach that was participative and empowering for all associated with it. In particular we tried to encourage those who Walker (1998) has referred to as having 'quiet voices' to 'have a say' in order to affect policy change at the local level. The most important input in the initiative therefore came from the full involvement of the project 'participants', and especially from the support and active engagement of Ying Wah Cheng, Norma Clarke, Pat Hadfield, Pam Haywood-Reed, Lilleth Millen, Movania Parkinson, Judy Robinson, Jean Wilkinson and Winnie Winfield. These nine women, all over 50 years of age and living in Sheffield, were recruited and trained to act as co-researchers on the project. Through the various levels of involvement, the project sought to explore the quality of life of older women, but also those possibilities for affecting change more widely through other locally based formal agencies.

Below we outline the nature of our research and the methodology involved, consider the academic and policy context relating to this research and focus upon the key findings relating to quality of life. We then suggest the main implications of our findings for policy and future practice. We are at an early stage of our analysis of the large quantity of rich data generated and our conclusions must at this stage remain tentative and be adjudged preliminary. The methodology we adopted and developed throughout the lifetime of the project should

149

inform the current 'modernising government' agenda and its encouragement of participative democratic involvement and the empowerment of citizens; even though this later concept remains contested and often abused (Starkey, 2003).

Objectives of the research

The central aim of the Older Women's Lives and Voices (OWLV) project was to demystify the lives of older women as a basis for change. This central tenet can be expanded into four key objectives:

1 To contribute to knowledge about older women's lives, especially their everyday understanding of quality of life.

2 To generate new knowledge about ways in which older women across different racial and ethnic communities promote their quality of life, particularly in relation to service use.

3 To inform policymakers and service providers about the experience of older women in using public services, defined as being relevant to quality of life and about older women's perceptions of their ability to 'have a say' about the services which impact on their lives.

4 To contribute to the development of ethically appropriate participatory or social action research methods in the study of policy and older women's lives.

Overarching these objectives, the primary focus of the research was to raise awareness of issues affecting the quality of life of older women across a range of different ethnic groups and their ability to have a say in services available to them. The study focused exclusively on initiatives within Sheffield and was aided, in part, by the involvement of one of the investigators in Sheffield's Better Government for Older People (BGOP) pilot network.

Background

Until recently there has been little focus within the UK on any broadly based qualitative research on the lives of older women, particularly those adopting a 'life story' approach. Where such work has been conducted, issues of identity and ethnicity have been marginalised and under-theorised (Bernard et al. 2000). The predominance of women in the population living to old age across Europe (Walker and Maltby 1997) means that a comprehensive analysis of the impact of social policy on the quality of life of older people needs to incorporate an understanding of the lives of older women. Older women from minority ethnic groups constitute an increasing proportion of this group as their statistical profile rapidly comes to mirror that of the white UK-born population (Schuman 1999: 33–43). It has been demonstrated that relative to older men, older women often report poorer levels of health (Jagger and Mathews 2002: 85–98) and lower levels of income (Ginn 2003), particularly when living alone. Indeed, many experience lengthy periods of chronic illness (Sidell 1995). However, few studies have directly explored the impact on the quality of women's lives of the intersection of age, gender and 'race' (Squires 1991), partly because of the relatively young profile of minority ethnic groups (Blakemore and Boneham 1993).

Our focus was on locally provided services, where recent policy has seen improving public and user participation as the mediator of a broader shift in the processes of social and public policy (Barnes 1997). Increased participation is not only intended to achieve more responsive and sensitive services, but also more legitimate and accountable public policies in light of the well-documented demographic shifts. Models for participation account for the factors above, rather than using them as excuses for excluding older people (Thornton and Tozer 1994; 1995; Knights and Midgley 1998). Examples include the Lewisham Older Women's Health Survey (Cooper and Siddell 1994) and the Fife User Panels Project (Barnes and Bennet 1997). Such approaches start from the experiences of older people themselves, rather than from the interests and concerns of the provider. They illustrate the importance of understanding not only how older women (and older people more generally) might be able to play a more active part in policy-making processes, but also the types of issues on which older women might want to have a say and what these imply for the practice of service professionals.

'Quality of life' is a contested concept and this research sought, through a qualitative and participative methodology, to ground it in an understanding of the lived experience of older women's lives from a range of ethnically diverse groups. Hence our use of the twofold delineation of quality of life as 'what factors are good and what makes life difficult'. Consequently, the measure we used was essentially descriptive and subjective yet allowed the participant at the personal level of analysis to reflect more broadly on those factors, in the past and present, which had affected their quality of life. This, we argue, can assist in refining social policy at the micro level and in turn lead to an improved quality of life for those women we have involved in our work.

Research design and methodology

The research built upon the methodology and findings from a pilot study of older women in Sheffield and Birmingham (Warren and Maltby 1998). The pilot used a life story approach (Plummer 1990), chosen for its potential to illuminate the 'inner' side of ageing (Ruth and Kenyon 1996) and to give people agency in defining their own needs, including self-supporting 'ordinary' older people (Hazan 1994; Bytheway 1997: 7–10).

The study built on the pilot in an organic way. That is, in order to be true to our participative approach we were open to changing intended approaches and to letting specific foci evolve as we found out more about the desires, needs and existing commitments of the women who took part. At the same time, the process raised important ethical concerns. The desire to link the new focus on individual human agency to the older focus on social structures of power and control (Hanmer and Hearn 1999: 106–30) underpinned the methodology of the project. As an exploratory rather than a representative project, we chose methods that had the main aim of encouraging the incorporation and active participation of older women.

Methodology and process

At the first stage of the project we ran 11 discussion groups with older women from existing social groups and political fora and each group met three times. Participants were encouraged to talk about the broad topics of 'growing older', 'using services' and 'having a say'. However, we left the interpretation of these phrases to them and the women were free to lead the discussion in whatever directions were important to them.

Ten volunteers were then recruited from the discussion groups and trained, through a series of workshops, to interview individual members of the groups in more detail about their lives and experiences. Working alongside the researchers, volunteers selected topics for and carried out these life story interviews as well as helping to identify what they saw as the main points of the findings. Over time, these ten volunteers were reduced to eight due to health reasons and the unanticipated death of Ying Wah Cheng. They all continue to play a key part in publicising these findings and associated recommendations for policy and practice through a number of seminars and talks to local service providers. Central to these stages was the production of a video featuring older women participants and documenting the project's development, findings and recommendations (Warren, 2003; LEMU, 2002).

We also wanted to allow an opportunity for individuals from the voluntary and statutory sectors involved in organising and providing services in Sheffield to air their views on the issue of participation in policymaking processes. Members of the project team interviewed 18 key people from a wide range of such agencies, asking them about schemes for increasing participation and their success in including older women (and older people) and widening the choices available to them.

All discussions and interviews were taped and transcribed for analysis. The analysis used the software package QSR Nud*ist to assist with the identification of the key themes and subthemes. The process is revealing commonalities and differences across the 11 discussion groups. It is also enabling the discovery of associations across all life stories, as well as across individual life stories and the discussions of the group within which individuals participated. Altogether, 100 women from black Caribbean, Irish, Chinese, Somali and white British communities participated in the project, though not at every stage. They were both users and potential users of services. Although not every participant had a record of their birth date, those who did indicated their ages ranged from 50 to 94 years with the mean being 68 years.

Recruitment to discussion groups was pragmatic and serendipitous (Warren et al. 2002) and needed to cap the number of potential communities involved to avoid diluting findings. Some groups were 'lost' as the result of local over-researching, compounded by our inability to guarantee changes to services. Links with other keen and relatively under-researched communities were made through personal contacts (including the project secretary) as well as via formal channels such as the Sheffield BGOP network.

The five communities provided us with the opportunity to look in depth at issues of disadvantage and diversity in older women's lives; for example, we were interested in black Caribbean women as independent recruits to the British workforce (Bhavnani 1994); Irish older women as members of the numerically biggest yet largely unrecognised minority ethnic group (Blakemore and Boneham 1993); Chinese older women as doubly excluded (for business reasons) from the mainstream economy and wider social participation; Somali women as very recent immigrants in the context of civil war (Brau 1996); and white British older women as the reference group against which understandings of the intersection of age, (female) gender and ethnicity are typically measured.

In the context of such diversity, negotiating the fine details of involvement often proved extremely 'labour intensive' (Cannon et al. 1991), even where access to groups was immediate. Repeated visits were required to build up trust with overworked and under-resourced community representatives, as well as the older women themselves (Lindow 1996). The pay-off was the increased confidence felt by participants when discussing issues. However, we found that members of some groups had never had the opportunity to share their experiences collectively before, which challenged our assumptions that association with a group necessarily implies inclusion.

Unsurprisingly, not all discussion group participants wanted or felt able to be involved in the research as volunteer interviewers for reasons of confidence, language, literacy, health, energy and alternative interests and commitments. The ten older women recruited, referred to collectively as 'the volunteers', came from a limited number of the more politicised groups and were amongst the younger and most vocal respondents in these groups and/or already active in public or voluntary roles. There was no volunteer from the Somali groups whose members uniformly were non-English speaking. Instead, members chose to be interviewed by one of the researchers working with an outside interpreter. This was the arrangement also for half of the life story interviews with members of the Chinese discussion groups as Ying Wah Cheng was the sole Chinese volunteer.

Despite these unforeseen events, a total of 44 life stories were gathered, the 'drop-off' being explained by deaths, illness and untranscribable tapes, rather than refusal. To prepare for interviewing, the volunteers took part in a series of workshops covering research design, interviewing, basic analysis, presentation and dissemination activities. The workshops were typically university based, half-day events, incorporating transport and lunch, and a small honorarium was paid for overall participation. However, here also, plans went through a series of revisions. The agenda for each workshop was invariably too ambitious and a number of extra workshops were necessary to cover everything fully.

Key findings on quality of life

Our analysis of the discussion groups is influenced by the nature of the data itself. As a result, themes are not easily separable and to avoid taking the data out of its context we have tended to analyse the issues as interconnected where it is useful to do so. The findings on quality of life and participation span all of the spheres of quality of life, including economic, socio-cultural participation, environmental resources and health. Here we focus on the following themes: the desire to have a say, the life experiences of older women and the positive aspects of growing older, and the opportunities and barriers to service provision and exercising agency. Within all these spheres the dynamics of gender, age and ethnicity are the key determinants to shaping not only the lived experience of growing older, but also the desire to have a say and the ability to get their views taken on board.

The desire to have a say

Despite the willingness of older women to become involved in the project and their enthusiasm for sharing their experiences, gathering data on the issue of agency was far from straightforward. We found that investigating abstract concepts like the 'quality of life' and 'the desire to have a say' required grounding in the issues that the groups raised themselves. Further, the group members came from a range of backgrounds and experiences. Some of them were used to expressing their views and active in lobbying service providers, while others had no experience of consultation. For many, the discussion group provided them with their first opportunity to discuss their experiences and needs collectively. Discussions of ageing and participation therefore were grounded in their experiences of services, ageism and the lack of recognition and targeted provision they felt their particular cultural group received.

The members were asked whether they 'felt listened to', 'are there things they would like to change', 'would they like to be consulted by service providers', 'what would encourage them to give their views'. Asking about 'having a say' in this way has generated some very rich material which contradicts the myth of older women as passive recipients of policy and services. For example, all of the women we worked with were keen to demonstrate their capacity to define their own needs and their determination to get their voices heard. Indeed, one of the fundamental findings of the project is that, when given the right support and opportunity, older women are more than capable of defining and expressing their own needs, and they have a strong desire to get their voices heard. One member who lived in a residential home stated:

> I am sure they thought I wish that old lady would go and lie down somewhere and shut up. I can't keep my mouth shut I have to say what I think, if they don't like it well I can't help it.
>
> (Irish participant in a mixed ethnicity group)

For many of the minority ethnic women the desire to have a say reflected the specific needs of that community group for culturally appropriate provision and targeted resources. One very active member of the Irish discussion group expressed this by saying, 'I am already out there shouting and making noises for and behalf of the Irish ... if I need to go and fall out with anybody then I will do it.' This participant's desire to push for the needs of her community was echoed in a lot of the discussion groups with minority ethnic women and is reflected in this quote by one Chinese group member:

> I do hope very much to have more of a say in government policy. So they would understand the needs of the ethnic minorities and provide appropriate services for us.

These findings demonstrate the desire of the women across the different groups to get their views heard and the effect that being listened to could have on their quality of life and access to services. As well as asking about 'the desire to have a say', the methods of this project inform the value of bringing older women together to discuss their experiences and needs. Perspectives on the value of participatory research varied across groups; for example, the four white British and one Irish group expressed an intrinsic value of taking part in the research. One Irish group member who had been a full-time carer for most of her life suggested:

> I feel a little isolated. This has been really uplifting to speak to somebody of my own age, somebody to understand what I am talking about ... It is so important, I have very good English friends but they wouldn't understand, the backgrounds are totally different.

The participatory approach was seen as a good way for the majority of those involved, to create space for the sharing and exchange of views with like-minded women who were not used to being asked their views. The following quote sums up the women's views on the general value of using open discussion groups:

> You see you starting life at 50, well most of the people have been brought up to accept things and not to complain against the system, or things like that, so you see getting into groups like this it can help to bring some people like that out.
>
> (White British group)

As the research progressed it became increasingly obvious that the degree to which the group members are excluded from services, particularly in relation to language difficulties, migration and racism, shaped what that particular group wanted to get from the research. This is not to say that white British and Irish groups were not keen for the research to have an impact, but the members of the Somali, Chinese and black Caribbean groups stressed to a greater degree, the importance of the research being used to raise awareness of their needs. Thus, the Somali and black Caribbean women cited instances where they had tried to get their views heard in the past and nothing had come of it. This resulted in many of them seeking reassurances from the research team that the project would be purposeful. One Somali group member expressed her frustration about the views of her group not being taken on board:

> We have been asked our views and needs in the past and nothing has changed. I have been living in this country for 12 years, discussing the same issues over and over again and nothing has changed.

The members of one mixed ethnicity group expressed their concerns that the views of older people were not taken seriously and were not used to implement change. These experiences were reflected by a member of the group from the black Caribbean community who stated:

> People get fed up of not being listened to and when you do get listened to, when you do lip service ... then they throw it in the bin ... They should work together [service providers and researchers] and listen and put practical things.

For the four groups we ran with Somali and Chinese older women, the issue of language and inadequate mainstream service provision heightened the importance of the research having an impact; for example, one Chinese group member requested:

> We hope that people like you [...] to tell what we want, we need a place of our own, we need funds to run the place, we need people like you to publicize so our voice can be heard, so we can get fund from the government.

The participants in this project felt that the route to a better quality of life lies in the ability to represent their own needs and for these needs to be taken on board in social policy and service planning. Key lessons can be derived from these findings. Not only do they demonstrate the importance of feeding back findings and outcomes to research participants and users, but also they illuminate some of the difficulties that service providers will face in encouraging user involvement and the need for them to implement these practices in a manner which takes account of past failures.

The life experiences of older women

Participants in many of the discussion groups recognised the stereotyping of older women as 'old biddies' or 'grannies' (Bytheway 1997: 7–10). A participant in her early fifties talked of being seen as an 'old woman' in her work as a business consultant and of the time taken to 'get through the barrier to show them that there is something worth listening to'. Yet ageing was not necessarily a negative experience for women. The gaining of experiences over time could lead to a growth in self-confidence and acceptance. Diminishing care responsibilities, as children grew up and left home, resulted in a greater sense of freedom to please themselves. Many participants articulated this as 'their time now to do what they want'. For most, this meant pursuing chosen activities post-retirement, including new educational, recreational and voluntary pursuits, though for a small number this applied to activities in paid employment.

The importance of family was common across all groups. Children may no longer have been dependent, but many women had taken on new caring roles as providers of childcare support for grandchildren, some to enable their daughters to take up career opportunities not open to themselves when they were younger. In this sense older women were important providers of support to their families, a role which they valued but that was not always based on choice for some participants. Other women were in a position where they were increasingly reliant on family members for practical, emotional and economic support. While this situation often involved rich and rewarding relationships with their families, some participants felt this eroded their independence and formed one of the negative aspects of ageing alongside others such as poor health and increasing disability and frailty, isolation and loneliness. This concern was reflected in the desires of participants to enter into dialogue with service providers to enable services to develop in a way that better met their needs and increased their independence.

In general, respondents across all groups found it difficult to manage on their income. Some had resorted to drastic measures such as selling possessions. Few Somali women received even a basic pension (not having been employed in the UK and without formal papers to prove their dates of birth they were reliant instead on Job Seekers Allowance). Women in this situation spoke of their subsequent loss of independence and sense of being a burden. Their forced dependence placed a strain on their families, while they in turn were coping with what they frequently saw as the breakdown of family traditions.

The obstacles to exercising agency

Participants expressed their concerns about the lack of consultation and involvement, and the desire and ability to define and express their own needs. In discussing their desire to be listened to they revealed several obstacles that make it difficult for them to voice their concerns and get their needs met by service provision. The majority of the women expressed the desire to be consulted on services and broader issues relating to their communities. However, when we asked them if they had ever been consulted or listened to, the common response was laughter. Few had experienced being asked their views or needs, and the overwhelming response was that they would welcome this opportunity but that it had to be followed up by real changes.

One of the overarching difficulties experienced by all of the women across the different groups was the ongoing barrier of ageism. As we have already noted, very few participants had experiences of voicing their individual views on policy issues. Stereotyping as well as past experiences could have the effect of limiting older women's lives and ambitions at both a cultural and structural level. For some participants it impacted on what they felt they were capable of doing. Some found it difficult in older age to believe that they still had something to offer and something worthwhile to say. For others, experiences of speaking out in the past had led them to become frustrated at not being listened to, and to feel disheartened with speaking out because nothing changed. For many participants, age discrimination had an impact on their everyday lives. One white British participant told of her experience with a GP:

> You are talking about age, this comes from a doctor, it makes you feel as though you are being patronised. ... I didn't know I had pneumonia. ... I said to him my friend says I have pneumonia. Do you know what he said 'we don't tell older people you got it in case it worries them'. That's so patronising.

Many of the women expressed the problems that ageism can pose and the following quotation from an Irish group member summarises how a large majority of them felt that their age resulted in their views being discounted:

> I know what I would like to get out of this [the research] is empowerment. Younger women are more able to take the power aren't they,

but for the older women it is sometimes very difficult, you feel you are discounted because you are no longer a chick.

Ageism was experienced to varying degrees by most of the women in our sample. However, the obstacles to services for minority ethnic women were far more dominated by the structural obstacles they experienced relating to language barriers, embedded racism and the failure of mainstream services to respond to their particular needs. For the Irish and black Caribbean women, their discussion of discrimination was often located in their past experiences of migration, education, health and work, and their ongoing experiences of racism more generally in their everyday lives. For many of the black Caribbean women racism has continued to permeate their experiences of health services and led to them receiving what they labelled as unequal treatment. Here we will focus upon the more overt experience of exclusion articulated by the Somali and Chinese women in the study. These examples demonstrate some of the more extreme difficulties that minority ethnic older women can face in accessing services, and thus they are a useful starting point for understanding the issues that shape quality of life in older age for these many ethnic minority women, and the importance of their participation in service decision making and research.

There is a marked difference in the way in which the Chinese and Somali groups described their experiences of services. The members of one of the groups of Chinese women were largely very satisfied with the services they received compared to what they would have received in mainland China or Hong Kong. Whereas both groups of Somali women were keen to stress their gratitude to the British government for giving them a home, they overwhelmingly felt:

> The government brought us here in UK but without appropriate provision of support and help. We do not know our rights.

The Somali women had migrated from a country where they felt able to easily access services and where they did not experience the same barriers to having their needs met. Moreover, they had come to Britain as refugees from civil war and felt that a lot of their treatment here was a result of discrimination as refugees, as well as a result of lack of understanding of their Muslim culture. In contrast, one of the Chinese groups felt generally that they had benefited from migrating to Britain, because service provision for older people was good compared to what they would have received in mainland China or Hong Kong:

> Since I am older, I am quite lucky to be living in England. Our welfare is quite well looked after by the government. Personally, I think I am fortunate. The government pay for all the services. When you're ill, there're health services which are very good.

However, the members of this group went on to illustrate areas where they felt services were insufficient. The second (younger) group of Chinese women held a very different perspective and spoke of the low expectations of services held by Chinese older people, for example, by saying:

> It's in our culture and we try to be self-sufficient and not to rely on others. Some of the older generation Chinese people don't want to ask for help.

Although half of the Chinese women felt happy with the welfare services they received, they faced many of the same difficulties as the Somali women. Some of these difficulties included poor access to translation services, inadequate information provision and awareness of rights, lack of community workers to help them access services, and inadequate understanding of their particular needs. Compared with the other ethnic groups involved in the study, the Chinese and Somali women experienced ageing from a very different starting point. Language barriers severely constrained their opportunities to participate more generally outside their local community group and to voice their concerns to bring about more inclusive service delivery. As a result, the majority of the women in these four groups expressed that language was the main barrier they experienced; it is what differentiates them from other older women. Language-based inequality can be seen as the root cause of their experiences of unequal treatment and discrimination.

Participants were keen to dispute the assumption often made by service providers that family members and friends will interpret for them. Many talked of their grandchildren missing school to translate for them and other family members not having good enough English to make their needs understood. Not only did the women cite several instances where they had tried to use services when interpreters were not provided, but they also raised concerns about the quality of interpreters when they are available. This extract from a discussion in one of the Somali groups reveals concerns over interpretation which, to a lesser degree, was also experienced by some of the Chinese women:

> Some of them call themselves professional interpreters but they lack the language proficiency ... Sometimes you feel sorry for some of the interpreters because you can see from their reaction that they cannot interpret to what is being said.

Participants often cited examples where language barriers alongside service providers' lack of understanding of their particular needs had made it extremely difficult for them to get the medical treatment they require, understand the treatment they are being given and access the benefits that they are entitled to:

> A lot of Chinese older women work hard all their lives. They're just like people of any other race, they can have physical illnesses and mental problems. But other people are able to seek help and support.

Many of the Somali women spoke of racism and communication problems:

> Sometimes you experience racism at some of the offices. You will be surprised the attitude of some of the staff ... the way they speak to you especially when your oral language is poor. You feel embarrassed ... I think this is disgusting and not acceptable and this actually discourages you when learning English language even if you are trying your best.

Disturbingly the Somali women, had experienced discrimination in relation to health services. The health issue is particularly important when we consider that many of the Somali women were affected by the civil war in their country and had lost loved ones, and were sometimes injured and had been deeply affected by the trauma of these events. All of the Somali women experienced communication problems with their GPs and other health professionals. Adding to this, the voluntary workers who support these women stated that there is not enough awareness of the physical and mental health needs of the Somali community in general that have resulted from their experiences of civil war.

The service providers' and policymakers' perspectives

The findings from our interviews with key personnel from various local statutory agencies and non-governmental organisations (NGOs) can be summarised in five points:

1 Raising expectations of those participating but also involvement leads to 'better' policy development.

2 There is a general lack of resources, both money and time. The message being conveyed was phrased more directly 'participation costs'!

3 The establishment of effective contacts, the development of trust and 'capacity building'.

4 Who participates? Is it only those who are (politically) involved or should agencies make greater efforts to capture the 'hidden voices', in our context the housebound or frail?

5 Finally, there was a small groundswell of opinion that indicated that research findings have not been acted upon and have not been a basis for change, which could lead to distrust and a lack of participation.

Such findings corroborate the work of Stevenson and Parsloe (1993) among others, which suggests that service providers and policymakers struggle with the challenges which user involvement has brought in terms of resources and organisational pressures. All such interviewees were keen not only to speak the language of modernisation (DoH 1998b) but also to act upon it. Yet often this keenness to incorporate a democratic participative approach to their professional practice was undermined by the underfunding of plans at local level together with pressures to meet national targets. Added to which, they each had their own set of priorities and needs combined with the difficulties of reaching what one of our respondents called the 'hidden voices' – those who are housebound, frail or too reticent or unable to become involved. In this respect, service providers and policymakers confirmed the long history of research being carried out that was not acted upon.

Although end users had often been consulted and involved, their expectations of change had been too high and often such expectations had not been realised as a result of political and financial pressure, as demonstrated in the analysis of the discussion groups outlined above. An issue that was reiterated throughout most interviews was the lack of financial resources and time to allow effective participation from 'service providers' and those end users. Clearly, participative methods may also not be part of everyone's agenda. The following quotation from a senior manager of a local NGO gives a flavour of these dilemmas:

> We have people coming to us and asking can we work with you now ... all things totally relevant to what we want to do, the strain for us is our resources. Our resources in becoming involved in that, it is really down to the director and myself because our other staff are working on specific projects ... The director and myself are also involved with regional work in [organisation name], the director is involved in national work in [organisation name], so it is quite stretching for us and very challenging.

Implications for social policy and policy research

This research has yielded both pragmatic outcomes for the development of research methodology as well as wider lessons for formulation and implementation of social policy. They have been identified jointly by the volunteers and the project team and contribute to what Barnes and Walker (1996) have referred to as a 'culture of empowerment' and have the potential to be extended to include all stakeholders and citizens and not simply older women.

Our work suggests that working in depth with a small number of groups provides greater insights into both quality of life issues and more importantly, allows those involved to give 'voice' to their concerns. Yet of crucial importance to the success of such strategies is the need to engage in extensive outreach work with communities to build trust, demonstrate a practical commitment to the issues and clarify aims and expected outcomes. 'Parachuting' into such communities suggests to that community or group that any outcome may be labelled 'lip service'. The provision of suitable venues and facilities for participants with disabilities and impairments and providing information that is both clear and understandable for everyone, for example, by use of 'plain English' is essential. So is the provision of experienced, adequately briefed and relatively independent interpreters and translators where second languages are involved. The provision of support, guidance, training and rehearsal for participation in any research and service decision-making processes and the valuing of the intrinsic benefits of involvement should also be considered. All this means that any such project should be adequately resourced, not only financially but also in the quantity and quality of time given to it.

In more general terms, our preliminary findings indicate the positive felt experience of growing older shared by the participants and their keenly felt desire to get their views heard in order to improve the meaning and quality of their lives, not only at an individual level but also for their peers.

9

Social support and ethnicity in old age

Jo Moriarty and Jabeer Butt

Introduction

The study of social relationships in old age has a long history in gerontological research. This can be seen from the classic studies such as those of Sheldon (1948), Townsend (1957) and Young and Willmott (1957) which were important landmarks in documenting the assistance given and received by older people (Phillips et al. 2000; Phillipson 1998a, 1998b). Since then, considerable attention has been given both to identifying those factors that enhance and hinder social support and to exploring the best ways in which it can be measured.

In relation to quality of life research, interest has broadly centred around the ways in which its presence or absence can contribute to an individual's quality of life and also, more specifically, on whether it lessens the potentially negative effects of events such as severe illness or bereavement (Helgeson 2003).

Although there is now an extensive body of work into quality of life, very little has been focused upon people from minority ethnic groups (Kart and Ford 2002; Nazroo et al. 2003). The implications of this gap are readily apparent. There has been a considerable increase in ethnic diversity within the population of the UK, largely as a result of immigration patterns during the 1950s and 1970s. This means that sampling strategies are required that reflect the ethnic diversity within the wider population. Researchers also need to consider whether the conceptual frameworks underpinning their research and methods of data collection are transferable across different ethnic groups. This is especially important within the context of the increasing interest in self-assessed aspects of quality of life which may be influenced by different cultural or socio-demographic characteristics (Kart and Ford 2002).

In this chapter we report on a study that aimed to examine quality of life and social support among older people from different ethnic groups. First, it summarises some of the existing literature relevant to this topic. Second, it describes the study methods and approach to collecting and recording information. Third, it discusses the key findings, highlighting some of the similarities and dissimilarities between different ethnic groups. Finally, it highlights their main implications for policy and practice.

What is meant by social support?

Social support is a broad term that includes all the supportive ways in which different people behave in the social environment (Helgeson 2003). While the terms 'social network' and 'social support' are often used interchangeably, a useful way of differentiating between the two has been provided by Bowling (1991) who used 'social network' to describe the set of people with whom one maintains contact and has some form of bond and 'social support' as the interactive process through which assistance is obtained from one's network. An alternative distinction can be made between network structure, which includes relatively objective measures such as the number of people within an individual's network and how they are related to him or her, and network function, which includes the exchange of social support in these relationships (Antonucci et al. 2001). The taxonomies of support described most often are:

- emotional – affection from others, sharing feelings or a general sense of belonging
- instrumental – tangible or material assistance, such as financial help
- informational – knowledge or advice provided by others (Newsom et al. 1997; Helgeson 2003).

Within these areas, a distinction is often made between subjective assessments of what is provided (perceived support) and the support that is actually provided (received or enacted support). Additional complexities are created when older people's social support is being studied because their relationships are often the product of many years of personal history and may span several generations (Antonucci and Akiyama 1987).

The relationship between social support and quality of life

Links between social support and quality of life have most often been presented in terms of the strong relationships that have been found between a person's social support and his or her physical and mental health. The two main arguments are based upon the buffering versus the main effects hypotheses. The first suggests that social support acts as a buffer. In the absence of stress or where it is minimal, social support and quality of life are unrelated. However, where a person undergoes stressful life experiences, good social support cushions against the impact of these difficulties. The second proposes that it has a main (direct) effect on health by increasing the sense of well-being and reducing vulnerability so that the more social support individuals have, the better their quality of life, regardless of their levels of stress (Cohen and Wills 1985; Gottlieb 1985; Moyer et al. 1999; Helgeson 2003). Network size, number of face-to-face contacts and the number of local ties are connected with the greater availability of practical and emotional support (Wenger and Tucker 2002). The presence of disability (for example, finding it difficult to leave the house) may lead to a reduction in the size of people's social networks and to changes in the types of support that are given and received (Ryan and Austin 1989).

Social support among older people in the UK

Work looking at older people's social support (for example Finch 1989; Qureshi and Walker 1989; Finch and Mason 1993; Arber and Attias-Donfut 1999) has emphasised both the strength of their ties and their complexities. It shows how relationships have been built up over time and are underpinned by a system of reciprocities and obligations. Economic and social changes have influenced the structures in which people provide and receive support, but there is no evidence that they are any more or less willing to do so. Furthermore, such changes do not automatically preclude the existence of continuities (Thane 2000).

Much of our knowledge about the social and support networks of older people in the UK is derived from the Bangor Longitudinal Study of Ageing (BLSA) which was based on a sample of 534 people aged 65 and over who were interviewed at five points in time between 1979 and 1991 (Wenger 1992, 1994, 1995; Burholt and Wenger 1998, 2001). Five main types of network (local family dependent, locally integrated, local self-contained, wider community focused and private restricted) were identified. The main differences between them related to the availability of local close family, the frequency of interaction within the networks, and the degree of involvement with the local community (Wenger and Tucker 2002). Individuals' networks were shaped by their marriage and fertility patterns, and those of their parents and grandparents, their migration history and that of their family and community, and by their personality. They were also subject to alteration as a result of changes in later life, such as bereavement or a decline in health (Scott and Wenger 1995).

Ethnicity and social support

Ethnic identity is a complex and dynamic concept encompassing ideas such as a shared past, language, identification with a specific religion and a distinctive culture (Blakemore and Boneham 1994; Fenton 1996). A small proportion of the published literature has examined how ethnicity or cultural background may influence social support. Classically, this has been presented in terms of individualistic versus collectivist societies (Hofstede 1980). At an individual level, people with gregarious personalities tend to report higher levels of social support and greater levels of satisfaction than individualist people who place greater emphasis on personal achievement and have higher reported levels of loneliness (Triandis 2001; Triandis et al. 1985, 1988).

What happens when individuals from one society move to a country where the majority of the population are from a different culture or ethnic background? Notwithstanding conceptual and methodological difficulties in the research, there is a growing literature, mainly North American in origin, on acculturation. This is the term generally used to describe what happens when groups of individuals of different cultures come into continuous contact, with subsequent changes in the original cultural patterns of either or both groups. Different strategies for adapting to these changes have been identified. Among the most well known is the fourfold model of integration, assimilation, separation and marginalisation (Berry 1992, 1997, 2001). While assimilation is widely agreed to be problematic because of its implicit assumption that the dominant culture is superior, limitations have also been identified in integrationist and multicultural models (Dominelli 1998). There is now increasing interest in models of biculturalism which argue that individuals are able to gain competence within two cultures without losing their cultural identity or having to choose one culture over the other (La Fromboise et al. 1993).

Social support plays a key role in understanding the processes that happen where societies are increasingly diverse because of the role of family, community and institutional ties in influencing how people adapt to these changes. On the one hand, existing attachments may be disrupted by migration. On the other, established members of a minority community may reach out to give support to newer arrivals. In some circumstances, comparatively high levels of social support among more recently established communities may act as a buffer against some of the stressors of being a member of a minority group, such as discrimination (Finch and Vega 2003). However, one of the difficulties in measuring social support in this context is the need to control for the potentially confounding effects of health status and immigration policies. For example, in the USA Latino immigrants, especially those whose legal status may be insecure, tend to have poorer health than the US-born population because their access to health care is poorer (Finch and Vega 2003). By contrast, in Canada where strict controls on the health status of potential immigrants exist, older people who have emigrated to Canada tend to have better health than the indigenous population (Wu and Hart 2002).

Existing studies looking at ethnicity and social support in the UK

A study based on interviews with 70 married couples originally from Gujarat who had moved to the Leicester area concluded that they had adopted successful strategies in which they maintained collectivist family values and a strong sense of identity but adapted some practices in line with prevalent norms within the white British community, such as greater acceptance that women might choose to have a career (Goodwin and Cramer 2002). Secondary analysis of the Fourth

National Survey of Ethnic Minorities (Modood et al. 1997) and qualitative interviews with a subsample of white British, black Caribbean, Punjabi Pakistani and Gujarati Hindu Indian respondents showed that although Punjabi Pakistanis generally had poorer health and lower incomes, their levels of social support and satisfaction with their neighbourhood were highest (Nazroo et al. 2003).

A multi-method study of white British, Asian Indian and Asian Bangladeshi older people undertaken in Woodford, Tower Hamlets and Wolverhampton (the same sites as those chosen by Sheldon 1948; Townsend 1957; Young and Willmott 1957) highlighted the importance of recognising the changing context in which people provide and receive support. It identified similarities between the dense kinship networks and multigenerational households found in Bangladeshi households in Tower Hamlets with those that had existed among white people in that district in the 1950s. On the whole, Asian Indian and Asian Bangladeshi participants were more likely than white people to have kin living locally. At the same time, there were also those for whom migration and poor health resulted in social isolation and experiences of loneliness. More positively, the majority of participants, whatever their ethnic background, did have someone in whom they could confide and who was able to help and support them. It also highlighted the uneven levels of knowledge about the support provided by statutory and voluntary organisations and the differences between those middle-class people who were confident in their ability to access services or arrange them themselves if necessary and poorer white and Bangladeshi participants who were often unaware of what help might be available (Phillips et al. 2000; Phillipson et al. 1998a, 1998b, 1999).

This last finding is consistent with other studies which have consistently shown that minority ethnic communities regularly have difficulties accessing those types of social support that are commonly provided by statutory agencies. These include instrumental social support such as help with personal care, or informational support such as advocacy (Ahmad and Atkin 1996; Butt and Mirza 1996; Katbamna et al. 1998; Ahmad 2000).

Study method

Data for the study was derived from semi-structured face-to-face interviews with a cross-sectional sample of 203 people aged 55 and over living in England and Scotland. The majority of participants (n = 101) were recruited from a sample of households who had participated in the Family Resources Survey (FRS), a nationally representative survey undertaken biennially on behalf of the Department for Work and Pensions (DWP). The total of 101 interviews represents 56 per cent of the original study population, 70 per cent of those we attempted to contact, and 76 per cent of those with whom we achieved contact. We increased the overall numbers of people from minority ethnic groups in the sample by recruiting people attending community centres or living in sheltered accommodation, resulting in a total of 68 people from seven different service settings. Lastly, we used snowball sampling through the interviewers' personal contacts (n = 34). Where the household consisted of more than one adult aged 55 and over, we attempted to interview all those aged 55 and over. This means that the final sample of 203 represents data from 173 households.

Interviewer matching and interview content

The majority of interviews were undertaken by a team of interviewers whom we had recruited and trained ourselves. Where possible we matched on the basis of ethnicity so that 74 per cent of white, 89 per cent of black, 98 per cent of South Asian, and all the Chinese participants were interviewed by someone of the same ethnic background.

The average interview lasted about an hour and a quarter (SD 28) and was undertaken in the participant's language of choice. Where permission was given, the interviews were recorded and the main open questions transcribed. A fifth of interviews took place in a language other than English and a further tenth used a combination of English and another language. They were translated into English by the interviewers, with the exception of the self-completion HRQoL questionnaire, the SF-36 (Ware and Sherbourne 1992) for which there was already a Chinese version, and versions of the SF-36 in South Asian languages which were specially prepared for use in this project. Although the majority of the interview was fairly structured, information on social support was collected in a more unstructured way. This was because existing instruments have been criticised for assuming that levels of social contact are indicative of the support available (Cordingley et al. 2001). We were also concerned that alternatives such as the Norbeck Social Support Questionnaire

173

(Norbeck et al. 1981) and the Lubben Social Network Scale (Lubben 1988) had not been validated in populations of people from different ethnic groups in the UK (Victor et al. 1999).

Information on social support

Our definition of a person's support network was broadly similar to that defined by Wenger (1984) as 'all those people with whom [a person] is in regular contact and who provide practical help, support and advice'. Using the past month as an initial reference point, participants were asked about the people that they saw or with whom they were in regular contact. We were interested in the:

+ *role* (partner, sibling, friend and so on)
+ *exchange* (what they did for one another and the nature of the relationship)
+ the *participant's perspective* of the interchange (for instance, satisfaction with the relationship, feelings of closeness).

Information on ethnicity

There is no consensus on what constitutes an ethnic group. Membership is something that is subjectively meaningful to the person concerned and the terminologies used to distinguish between groups have changed markedly over time (ONS 2002b). Participants were asked to self-identify their ethnic group from the list of categories used in the 2001 English Census and we used the same output categories recommended for National Statistics data sources. Britain's minority ethnic populations have different age structures, reflecting past immigration and fertility patterns. Therefore, where numbers are too small to be presented by ethnic group we sometimes combine different categories. We also use the terms 'South Asian' or 'black' where more specific details might lead to individual participants being identified.

Characteristics of the sample

Consistent with the age structure of Britain's minority communities, Black Caribbeans and Asian Indians comprised the largest proportion of study participants from a minority ethnic group. They each represented 27 per cent of the sample as a whole and 34 per cent of participants from a minority ethnic group. Thirteen participants defined themselves as Asian Pakistani and the remainder consisted of Chinese people (11), Black Africans (7), Asian Bangladeshis (5) and people from other ethnic groups or of mixed heritage (17). Just under a fifth of participants were white (38). The mean age of the sample was 69 (SD 8), with Asian Bangladeshi and Black African participants being younger than their white British, Black Caribbean and Asian Indian counterparts, as was to be expected given their differing age structures (ONS 2002a). The sample was almost equally divided between men and women. The geographical distribution of people from minority ethnic groups broadly reflected their distribution within the population as a whole in that the majority were concentrated in London, the Midlands, or the North-West (ONS 2002b).

Main findings

Social support as an important constituent of quality of life

The overwhelming majority of participants, whatever their ethnicity or gender, were in regular contact with members of their family and friends. Almost two-thirds were married or living with a partner. Very few were single and almost all the remainder were widowed or divorced. Levels of childlessness were low in that 93 per cent had one or more living children.

Thirty-one per cent of participants described an aspect of their lives relating to their relationship with their family as something that made their life good. This is consistent with another study in which 31 per cent of people rated their relationships with their family and relatives as the most important thing in their life in priority order (Bowling 1995a). A widowed white British man explained:

[The most important thing in my life] is the love of my family ... It's the contact with the family and also with, you know, friends that makes life really worthwhile.

In contrast to men who were more likely to mention good health or an adequate income before social support, women were more likely to attach greatest importance to their social relationships:

[Laughing] Do I have to mention [name of husband who was present in the room]? Well, first family and living in peaceful surroundings, I mean that's about the best isn't it? And you could say, fairly good health.

(White British woman)

For others, there was a stronger interrelationship between social support, health and quality of life. A black Caribbean woman had always felt well supported by her children and members of her church but they had increased their contact when she was ill:

The hospital was packed, plenty people couldn't come and even see me. And when I'm sick at home and they know that I'm sick, the house is packed. The children come right down and so forth ... [What is good about my life is] to know that I have a very strong family background, both with my children, their friends and my friends, and my brothers and sisters [i.e. fellow church members].

Impact of migration

Given the broad agreement among all participants, whatever their ethnic background, about the importance of social support in contributing to quality of life, how might it have been affected by moving to a different country? With two exceptions, all the participants from a minority ethnic group had been born outside the UK whereas just two white participants had been born elsewhere. However, given that the mean length of UK residence was 36 years (SD 12), the majority of participants from a minority ethnic group had lived longer in the UK than in their country of birth, as many of them pointed out.

Sixty-two per cent of men from a minority ethnic group had moved to the UK to take up paid employment, 14 per cent to undertake further education, and 12 per cent to join their family. By contrast, 66 per cent of women came to join their families, 18 per cent to find paid employment and none to undertake further education. This meant that while men had tended to rely upon social contacts established through the workplace, women's were more centred on their family.

There were also differences between ethnic groups in that 'chain migration' in which several members of the same family moved at or around the same time was more common among Asian Indian, Asian Pakistani and Asian Bangladeshi participants. Many had settled in geographically close proximity to each other and their local networks often included kin such as siblings, sisters or brothers-in-law, and nieces and nephews. By contrast, among Chinese, Black African and Black Caribbeans, such kin were likely to live further away or outside the UK altogether.

Changes to immigration, citizenship, and asylum laws from the 1970s onwards have restricted the number of people eligible to move to the UK. Fourteen participants had moved as a result of political instability in their country of birth. These included East African Asians and people who had arrived as asylum seekers. For them, the process had been more difficult, as one man explained:

> I was about 45–50 years old and I leave behind me many many relatives, many many friends, my background, my culture. Yes, I was free politically and economically but mentally I wasn't free ... because my heart was still there ... It was difficult, very very difficult when I came to make friends because at that time there were very few Kurdish people here [and] because I couldn't speak any English at that time.

However, since his arrival he had re-established friendships with people he had known in Iraq, was in regular telephone contact with family and friends living outside the UK, and had established new friendships that included some of his white neighbours. On the whole, this pattern was very typical. It was noticeable how quickly people had begun to rebuild their social support upon arrival in Britain, often showing considerable adaptability.

Sometimes they proactively began to rebuild their support even before their arrival by moving to areas in which they already had family or friends (pull factors), a pattern that has also been observed in Canada (Wu and Hart 2002). Once in the UK, people had tended to settle quickly into one area. At 26 years (SD 14), the mean length of residence in their locality among people from minority ethnic groups was shorter than that for white participants (41, SD 23), but was still considerable. Levels of satisfaction with their neighbourhood were extremely high with access to shops, places of worship and public transport being cited as among the main advantages, a finding that has been reported elsewhere (Nazroo et al. 2003).

Types and sources of social support

Across all ethnic groups, there was a marked difference between participants who described systems that were 'rich' in terms of the breadth and depth of their social support and those that were more restricted. The former tended to be well integrated into their local community, had comparatively high household incomes, reported better self-rated health and fewer specific health problems, and could be seen as net providers of support in the sense that they provided more support than they received. By contrast, those with more restricted support tended to have lower incomes, poorer health and had few relationships beyond their immediate family. Even these relationships were often reported as being problematic. Nevertheless, although social support was influenced by structural determinants such as poor health and lack of income, different participants responded to these barriers in different ways. For example, one woman felt that 'I can't do my own things so how can I help others?' However, another woman who was housebound saw this as no barrier to regular visits from friends to whom she was 'an agony aunt'.

Beyond this broad pattern, some differences between different ethnic groups did emerge. Although close proximity to children does not imply frequent contact, it does have implications for the sort of support that can be provided in that while emotional support might be provided through telephone calls and email, regular practical assistance or help in an emergency is less easy to provide (Shelton and Grundy 2000).

Including co-resident children and children living within a 20-mile radius, over 90 per cent of South Asian participants had at least one child living locally. They were the group in which an intensive routine of support systems were described most often. Instrumental support, usually provided by daughters or daughters-in-law in the form of cooking, shopping or cleaning was reciprocated, usually by looking after grandchildren. Children tended to visit their parents, rather than the reverse. Friendship networks were local and mainly included neighbours and people who had migrated at the same time or whom they had known in their country of birth. On the whole, these friendships were used for socialising rather than to provide emotional support. Although traditionally there has been an assumption that daughters would join their husband's family (Ahmad 1996), the majority of women looked to blood relationships rather than relationships by marriage for emotional support and often described close relationships with daughters or sisters. For some topics, such as concerns about health, a sister or daughter was the preferred confidante to their husband. Men often looked outside the family to contacts made through community faith-based or welfare organisations and, occasionally, through local councillors for informational support. Although wives and friends of their own age or older could be a source of emotional support, some South Asian men felt that it would be inappropriate for them to discuss problems with those who were younger:

> You see, I'm the older one. I can't talk about my problems. I listen to other people's problems.
>
> (Asian Pakistani man)

Although levels of practical and emotional support were high, their provision was often reliant upon just one or two family members. This was demonstrated in the interviewers' ratings of participants' support. These suggested that only a third of South Asian women and just over a half of South Asian men had multiple sources of support.

While caution must be taken in view of the small numbers involved, it seemed that the trend towards greater geographical distances between parents and children among those with higher levels of education and employed in professional jobs observed in white communities (Shelton and Grundy 2000) was discernible among the families of Asian Indian and Asian Pakistani participants from professional or managerial and intermediate occupations.

Eighty-four per cent of black Caribbean and mixed white and black Caribbean participants had at least one child living locally. Here, the pattern whereby in larger families one child remains in close geographic proximity to the parent(s) but others are more dispersed (Shelton and Grundy 2000) was most apparent. Contrary to some stereotyped assumptions, a high proportion of black Caribbean older people live on their own (Lowdell et al. 2000), and almost half of the black Caribbean households participating in the study consisted of one person. Although they frequently reported that their health was poor and their incomes tended to be lower than other participants, their levels of social support were generally high. In some cases, the closeness of their relationships had been increased through support at times of illness or a shared religious faith. It was noticeable that their networks were almost equally divided between family members and close friends, often made through the church or local community centre. In addition, many had kept in touch with friends who had emigrated from the Caribbean to the USA or Canada and described regular contact through visits or holidays. Based on the interviewers' ratings, 75 per cent of black Caribbean men and 80 per cent of women had multiple sources of support.

On average, white people had fewest children and they, along with Chinese people, were least likely to have at least one child living within a 20-mile radius. This may partly explain why they were more likely to look to their children for support in a crisis (Harper 1987), rather than to provide regular assistance. Irrespective of gender, white people were more likely to report having two or more confiding relationships than any other ethnic group. Although this information was collected in an unstructured way so it is possible that they were simply more likely to choose to report it than other ethnic groups, it may be that they set more importance upon emotional support than other forms of assistance. Friendship networks consisted of local and distant friends and, where participants were married or living with a partner, distinctions were often made between those who were joint friends and those who were closer to one partner. Around three-quarters of white men and white women were rated by the interviewers as having multiple sources of support. In many cases, this reflected an embeddedness in their local communities through many years of residence or through active attempts to rebuild their social networks following a move to another area on their retirement.

On the whole, participants from other ethic groups tended to have smaller networks, both of kin and of friends. This was related to multiple factors, such as having arrived here at a comparatively old age in the case of refugees, being a member of a minority group that was small in size or geographically dispersed, or because they had emigrated since the application of stricter immigration rules and other family members had to remain in their country of birth.

Caring relationships

The existing literature (Qureshi and Walker 1989; Arber and Ginn 1991; Wenger 1992; Parker and Lawton 1994) makes clear that instrumental support in the form of help with shopping or cleaning may be provided from within a wider network of friends and neighbours but that personal care, such as assistance with washing or dressing, is overwhelmingly provided by spouses or other household members. However, it is often assumed that people from minority ethnic groups can rely on extended families for support (Katbamna et al. 1998; Social Services Inspectorate 1998). In this study, 41 participants were providing unpaid care for an older person or person with disabilities. While this number is too small to permit generalisations on the basis of ethnicity, the overall picture was consistent with other work suggesting that carers from South Asian communities did not receive extensive support from other members of their family and friends (Katbamna et al. 1998). South Asian carers were more likely to provide care within the household whereas black Caribbean and white participants provided support inside and outside the household. For white widowed and single men, driving friends or neighbours to the shops or appointments or carrying out household repairs was sometimes a way of accessing support of their own.

Black Caribbean carers often described providing support to more than one person and, among those who were church members or who attended community centres, the patterns of support were similar to those among African-Americans where caring networks tend to be larger and less likely to consist solely of spouses and adult children (Janevic and Connell 2001; Williams and Dilworth-Anderson 2002).

Support from health and social care services

Since the earliest studies in which older people's support from health and social care services was compared with so-called informal help from family, friends and neighbours (Litwak 1985; Chappell and Blandford 1991; Chappell 1992), the balance between the two has been shown to be very strongly in favour of the latter, except in cases of very severe disability. Consistent with this picture, only a minority of participants received support from health and social care services.

We collected details on the use of 11 health and social care services, excluding GPs (home care, day care, meals, lunch clubs, community nurses, community psychiatric nurses, social workers, occupational therapy, physiotherapy, chiropody, and welfare rights and benefits), using non-technical descriptions as well as their official titles, as advised by other researchers (Mark Johnson and Savita Katbamna, personal communications). Just under half the sample were neither using, nor had ever used, any of these services. Among these, it is important to emphasise that three-quarters were happy with this situation and felt that such services were currently unnecessary. However, a quarter (n = 30) said that they would like to try one or more service, with the one most requested being welfare rights and benefits (n = 11). Given that over a third of pensioner households for which we had information had incomes less than the current minimum income guarantee of £102.10 a week for a single person or £155.80 a week for a couple, it is arguable that the need for such a service extended beyond this subgroup.

Among those aged 65 and over, 18 per cent were using chiropody, 14 per cent home care, 2 per cent used a meals service and 3 per cent had seen a social worker. These are broadly similar to the proportions reported in the *1994 General Household Survey* among this age group (Bennett et al. 1996). Figures for attendances at day centres or lunch clubs are much higher (22 and 13 per cent respectively) but this is undoubtedly an artefact of sample selection. Overall, the mean number of services used was one (SD 1.6) although, as was to be expected, it was higher among those recruited via sheltered housing and community centre settings (mean 2, SD 2). However, these levels of service use are not high, especially when the overall levels of reported disability within the sample are taken into account. For example, the *2001 General Household Survey* reported that 37 per cent of people in the 65 to 74 age group and 46 per cent of those aged 75 and over had a longstanding illness or disability (Walker et al. 2002). In this sample, the equivalent proportions were 63 and 80 per cent. Furthermore, the use of privately arranged services to substitute or complement publicly funded ones was rare, with just 11 per cent of those aged 65 and over employing either a handy person, cleaner, or care assistant.

Using the same list, participants also provided information about the services that they had known about prior to the interview. Forty-three per cent had heard of them all but levels of awareness were higher among white British and Black Caribbeans. In the case of the latter, as they themselves pointed out, many of them had acquired this knowledge through paid employment in health and social care. Other ethnic groups appeared to be less familiar with these services and this seemed to be related to the ability to speak English, highlighting the difficulties for those unable to access publicity only made available in English.

Support from voluntary organisations

Almost without exception, the only participants who included contacts made through voluntary organisations in their social networks (as distinct from faith-based, sporting or social clubs) were the subsample of South Asian, Chinese and black Caribbean participants (n = 68) who were recruited via community centres and sheltered housing schemes run by voluntary organisations aimed at supporting people from minority ethnic groups. Compared with other participants, these people were less likely to be currently married and more likely to live on their own. They tended to have fewer confiding relationships but more people providing practical help.

They tended to use support from voluntary organisations in different ways. Some had networks that resembled the diffuse tie networks described among Russian Jewish emigrés to Israel (Litwin 1995) in that their networks were comparatively large but contained few close ties. Face-to-face contact with family members was often limited and the majority of their social lives took place in lunch clubs, day centres, or community centres. A Chinese woman explained: 'I don't know their names. I just say "hello" to them.' By contrast, others arranged attendance at centres around help from their family, visiting them on days when they did not see their children.

For those who did not speak English, voluntary organisations were an especially vital gateway to other forms of help. In some cases, workers would translate official letters for them or put them in touch with interpreters. In other cases, they arranged for health and social care professionals to visit the centres on a sessional basis or they accompanied participants to appointments. A Chinese couple explained: 'If we're ill or need to go the dentist or the opticians, we tend to ask the staff that work at the Community Centre [to accompany us].' Voluntary organisations could also be a source of more intimate emotional support. In one centre for black Caribbeans, nearly all the members had originated from the same area in Jamaica. Their relationships had been established over many years and in some cases were based upon frequent levels of contact in that they socialised outside the centre and attended the same church.

Satisfaction with and expectations about support

Consistent with the literature, women were more likely to be satisfied with their social support than men, with 85 per cent of women and 70 per cent of men being satisfied. Levels of satisfaction were related to the presence of two or more confiding relationships rather than to whether or not participants were in contact with members of their family, friends and neighbours, suggesting that what was important was not the quantity of social contacts, but their quality.

An important issue is the extent to which satisfaction with social support and quality of life was related to expectations. This is a notoriously difficult area to explore, partly because beliefs about normative behaviour may overlap across ethnic groups, as well as being influenced by other factors such as gender, age and occupational background (Ahmad 1996) and partly because there is not always a direct relationship between normative beliefs and action (Finch and Mason 1993). Indeed, one of the clearest examples where contrasts between normative beliefs about what should happen and practical responses to actual situations could be seen among participants who were carers where, for example, five South Asian men were providing considerable amounts of care.

Another area where differing expectations and ideas about perceived support impacted on quality of life emerged in views about the help that might be expected from children. First of all, it is important to recognise that many participants directly related their own quality of life to that of their children's: 'I am a traditional Chinese woman. It makes me happy to see all my children with a nice future, good jobs and family themselves.' Although this participant made reference to her ethnicity, it was an attitude shared by participants from other ethnic groups and provided an example where participants sometimes ascribed certain values to their ethnicity when the views expressed by others suggested that it was a value either shared across ethnic groups or an individual preference. For the majority of participants, the interconnecting of parental and children's quality of life was a source of pride and pleasure. For a minority, it was a potential source of conflict if children appeared to choose a lifestyle that did not conform to their parents' expectations.

Second, the degree to which participants were satisfied with the support from children seemed to depend upon the extent to which they differentiated between the 'ideal' and what was feasible:

> You cannot blame the youngsters. They are very busy in this country ... [and] they've got to look after their children as well and they haven't got time to look after old people so I don't blame them.
>
> (Asian Indian man)

By contrast, another person received high levels of actual support from her daughter. However, she compared herself unfavourably with other people who had been 'blessed with good children' and, although she had been provided with home care after a stay in hospital, she decided to cancel it and move in with her daughter temporarily. In her eyes, the support she received from a day centre and her neighbours was automatically inferior to support from children.

Discussion

The importance of social support as a constituent of quality of life was an idea that was widely shared across all participants, whatever their ethnic group. Although attention needs to be paid to ensuring that the structural determinants of social support such as access to health care and an adequate income are in place, acknowledgement should be made of the resourcefulness shown by individuals and the active steps that they took in shaping the framework for their social lives. It was very striking that in a sample in which levels of self-reported health tended to be poor and household incomes were comparatively low, levels of social support were so high.

At the same time, the study also suggested that there were areas in which individuals could be assisted to improve their social support. In this age group, the majority of people from minority ethnic groups have not been born in the UK. The process of migration is a change agent in itself, affecting people's roles, expectations and reciprocities (Ahmad 1996). Participants' accounts of the circumstances in which they had moved to the UK suggested that the ways in which social support is affected on migration are likely to be the result of a complex series of interactions that include gender, reason for moving and the legal framework governing entry to the 'receiving' country. However, the extent to which these changes become permanent are influenced by individuals' own sense of agency, by the extent to which they are able to access support from other members of their ethnic group, and the degree to which they feel they have been accepted by the 'receiving' community. In this sense, the act of migration is unlikely to have a long-term negative effect on people's social support. What will have an effect is if they become socially excluded through not being given opportunities to share fully in the economic and social resources of the 'receiving' country.

Furthermore, what was true of those who emigrated in the 1960s and 1970s may not be true for other groups. On the whole, participants who had emigrated earlier, generally for reasons of employment or as spouses, had better social support than those who arrived later as asylum seekers and refugees. While firm conclusions cannot be drawn from so small a subgroup as those included in this study, it suggests that there is a need for further work examining whether different patterns of migration have an impact upon patterns of ageing and possible future care needs (Blakemore 1999).

The study highlighted the need for greater appreciation of the differences between and within different ethnic groups (see also Chapter 3). For example, on the whole, Chinese people are more geographically dispersed than other minority ethnic groups and in the older age group have often worked in occupations where long hours have limited their opportunities to build up extensive support networks. Asian Indian and Asian Pakistani participants who had professional and managerial backgrounds showed greater similarities with their white counterparts.

In the same way, the need to separate out different components of social support was also made clear. The study showed the substitutability of the provision of instrumental support in the form of help with shopping or cleaning. Among South Asian communities, such tasks were generally undertaken by children; among white people, by neighbours or friends; among black Caribbeans by children or friends. However, across all ethnic groups, as the literature on caring in white communities has shown so forcefully, personal care was almost always provided by close relatives, most often spouses. This highlights the need not to assume that those living in multigenerational households or who have local kin will automatically have access to additional support as carers (Katbamna et al. 1998). Findings from the study also suggested that in some ethnic groups there may be more tightly defined rules about the sharing of emotional or personal problems, highlighting the need for health and social care providers to become 'culturally competent' (Betancourt et al. 2003).

Through the *National Service Framework for Older People* (DoH 2001) and the *Fair Access to Care Initiative* (DoH 2002), the government has emphasised that people with similar levels of need should expect to receive the same sort of services, whatever their background and wherever they live. Given the high prevalence of disability, access to health and social care services seemed to be comparatively low. The low levels of service utilisation among people from minority ethnic groups has been a recurring theme (Ahmad and Atkin 1996; Butt and Mirza 1996; Ahmad 2000) and this study showed that it remains a cause for concern.

Government policy has also highlighted the potential role to be played by faith-based and community organisations (Smith 2003). Black voluntary sector and ethnically based community organisations are often viewed as means for reinforcing bonds among minority ethic group members through, for example, providing opportunities to share food and festivals. However, our study suggested that their role bridging between minority ethnic groups and mainstream organisations should be extended. This is particularly important for people who do not speak English who are often extremely reliant upon the informational support they receive from workers in such organisations.

Finally, the study suggests that further work should focus on perceived as opposed to actual social support. This would contribute to the growing literature on the impact of expectations on perceptions of quality of life (Higgs 1999; Selai et al. 1999; Carr et al. 2001; Bowling et al. 2002).

10

The meaning of grandparenthood and its contribution to the quality of life of older people

Lynda Clarke and Ceridwen Roberts

Introduction

At the end of the 1990s there was a sudden upsurge of popular and policy interest in grandparents. The ageing of the population meant that never before had so many people lived long enough to become grandparents and the grandparent–grandchild relationship had become more prevalent as a result of demographic changes in child-bearing patterns and the age structure of the population. Popular views of the extended family as a thing of the past were increasingly super-seded by a policy view that welcomed the practical role that older people could play either as grandparents, supporting their own children in the care and upbringing of their grandchildren, or as people active in the community working with the young. This view is epito-mised in the Labour government's key family policy document *Supporting Families* (Home Office 1998), which recognised that grandparents can and do play important caring roles in the lives of many children and asked how government could encourage grand-parents to be involved in their grandchildren's education and in supporting parents. At the same time the government's Better Gov-ernment for Older People initiative was attempting to look at the reality of older people's lives and challenge the stereotypical thinking that underlay much public provision for and attitudes towards older people (Shreeve 2000).

Yet it could be argued that there was a tension here as much of the public and policy discourse around the role of grandparents at this time was characterised by an unthinking assumption of homogeneity and by an approach which saw grandparents as a resource for others rather than as people in their own right with complex wishes and family situations. Moreover, at the point at which arguments about the importance of grandparents were being presented in public policy, there was no available national information in Britain about the prevalence of grandparenthood or the diverse family and socio-economic circumstances in which grandparents performed out their roles and the meaning they attached to them (Clarke and Cairns 2001; Clarke and Roberts 2002).

This project planned to test these assumptions and set out to both 'map' the characteristics of older people's entry into grandparenthood, the degree of contact they had with their children and grandchildren, the activities they undertook as grandparents and, most importantly, to explore with older people who were grandparents what being a grandparent meant and whether this role or status contributed to or detracted from their quality of life.

Grandparents and family life: the evidence and the issues

There had been little British research on grandparents since the classic works on kinship of Townsend, Willmott and Young in the 1950s and 1960s which revealed the centrality of the mother–daughter relationship. Subsequent survey data in the 1980s and 1990s confirmed the continuing emotional and/or practical importance of grandparents within the three generation family (Martin and Roberts 1984; Willmott 1986; Finch 1989; McGlone et al. 1998) but there was almost no research in Britain which considered the experience of becoming and being a grandparent from the point of view of older people themselves. Until recently, what we knew about grandparents was drawn from a few qualitative studies focusing on specific issues and some quantitative work on older people and kin exchanges from a general perspective. Such studies included work on becoming a grandparent, negotiating the grandparental role in the family, grandfatherhood and grandparents' material help for families with young children. (Cunningham-Burley 1985, 1986, 1987; Wilson 1987). Finch and Mason (1993) also undertook both a survey and a qualitative examination of family obligations and responsibilities which included grandparents.

More recently in the 1990s, a number of studies, although not investigating grandparenthood directly, have provided useful insights on the social life and kin support of older people in certain locations or for particular groups of people. Some evidence of grandparental input into families can be gleaned from questions on patterns of contact and support from extended family members, for example, the British Social Attitudes Survey (BSAS) kinship module of 1995 (McGlone et al. 1998) and a module on young people in the 1998 BSAS included grandparenting, but only from the grandchild's perspective. These studies have all provided useful clues about specific facets of being a grandparent, but were not designed to be generalised or aimed at exploring the grandparental role in particular. Other work relevant to grandparenting and family change has been done by demographers in the area of describing, analysing and modelling family breakdown and household composition (for example, Clarke 1992; Clarke et al. 1997; 2000). Changes in the age structure of the population and the level of family change are highly relevant in determining the availability of kin, but they do not provide any information about how such relationships operate nor their meaning to the individual concerned.

Several studies have given us insights into how older people's lives and expectations have changed over the last decades. Phillipson et al. (1998b) returned to the urban areas of the three major studies of older people in the 1940s and 1950s (Bethnal Green, Wolverhampton and Woodford) to examine the change and continuities in the lives of older people. He found that kinship ties remained central to these older people but that they were more likely than 50 years ago to live alone and to have important 'personal communities' in the shape of friends.

The impact of family change on older people has also been examined in a qualitative study, on intergenerational ties and transfers in stepfamilies (Bornat et al. 1998). This study found that family break-up and reconstitution brings some older people, their adult children and stepchildren closer together but may lead to older men living in relative isolation, while ties between mothers and daughters may be strengthened. Another small-scale study assessed the impact of divorce on the grandparent–grandchild relationship. This showed that grandparents who reported a loss of contact with grandchildren had emotional and physical health problems related to this loss. It provided valuable insights into the effect of separation or divorce on grandparents but was limited, however, as the sample of grandparents was small and self-selected (Drew and Smith 1999).

Studies exploring the meaning of the experience of grandparenthood for older people, however, have been much rarer, although one by Age Concern (1998) which explored the role grandparents felt they played in the lives of their grandchildren confirmed that this role was important for many older people in Britain. Another qualitative study examined the negotiation of the grandparental role within the family (Tunaley 1998). It showed that while grandparents played an active role in their families, both parents and grandparents asserted that they should not 'interfere' in their children's and grandchildren's lives.

It was not until the late 1990s that nationally representative data on household and family structure became available which provided a picture of the prevalence and nature of modern grandparenting. Research investigating kin exchange beyond the household by Grundy et al. in 1997–8 established a framework of all kin exchanges, including grandparental exchanges. Their nationally representative study pro-vided the first national data on the prevalence of grandparenthood showing, for example, that 44 per cent of 50 to 59 year olds and 71 per cent of 60 to 69 year olds in 1997–8 were grandparents (Grundy et al. 1999).

The picture was taken further by the 1998 BSAS (Dench et al. 1999) which represents a first specific look at grandparenting using a nationally representative sample. The survey module asked grand-parents about their relationship with one randomly selected grandchild and vice versa. Most of the respondents regarded their relationships with their grandchildren as extremely important and 64 per cent of the grandparents agreed that 'grandparenting is a very rewarding aspect of my life'. The survey provides a general and valuable overview of atti-tudes towards various aspects of the grandparenting experience, but inevitably because of its structured nature could not look in depth at any one issue.

What was known from a social science perspective, therefore, about the grandparent–grandchild relationship came chiefly from research in the USA where interest in grandparent–grandchild and grand-parenthood was much more extensively developed (Silverstein and Marenco 2000). This research demonstrated that for many older people family links and intergenerational solidarity may be crucial in contributing to the quality of many older people's lives and for the avoidance of social exclusion among older people. The relationship with grandchildren is an important adjunct therefore to their relationship with spouses and their children. Indeed relationships with grandchildren may become increasingly important for grandparents as they get older. Their spouse may die or exit from their lives and relationships with children and grandchildren may be renegotiated as the balance or type of dependency changes.

In a recent study of quality of life, relationships with family and relatives were most frequently named as the most important thing in current life, well ahead of any other aspect (Bowling 1995b). These relationships then encompass emotional, practical and financial support as well as less tangible feelings of mutual support and reciprocal obligation. Intergenerational exchanges, however, work in both directions (Qureshi and Walker 1989; Aldous 1995) and where both parents are working or where family breakdown has occurred, grandparents may be expected to care for grandchildren or to contribute to their support in financial or emotional terms. McGlone et al. (1998), for example, revealed that grandparents play an important role in the lives of families with young dependent children. However, there is a potential for tension here if grandparents' wishes and capacities for involvement and support and the needs and expectations of their children and grandchildren for grandparental help are not kept in balance. It is likely that this tension has increased over the 1990s for a variety of reasons. With increasing numbers of mothers being encouraged to return to employment throughout the 1980s and 1990s there has been a higher demand for childcare and much of this demand, especially for the non-professional classes, is being met by grandparents as historically has been the case. Equally levels of family break-up have increased and this has been occurring earlier in the life of a relationship so children are often quite young when their parents separate. At the same time, older people are not only living longer, but are also living healthier lives for longer. As attitudes change towards older people's independence and autonomy, supporting their families may be at odds with their own desires or indeed need to continue in paid employment or pursue other leisure interests after a working life.

Aware of how the world of both grandparents and parents had changed over the last decades, our investigation was focused on exploring the diversity of grandparents' family circumstances and their activities. We were particularly interested in whether family changes and breakdown or changes in proximity had affected grandparents and to what extent being a grandparent was an important source of identity for older people and contributed to their sense of well-being and worth. Did it contribute to the quality of their lives?

American analysts have identified five major dimensions of social differentiation in grandparenting roles: across historical time; between men and women; between older and younger individuals; among ethnic and subcultural groups; and between individuals as grandparents (Bengtson and Robertson 1985). More recently, the number of sets of grandchildren, age of the grandchild, marital status of the grandchildren's parents, social class, education and income have all been identified as other major determinants in styles of grandparenting (Silverstein and Long 1998; Uhlenberg and Hammil 1998). These studies have also indicated that where contact is infrequent this is often as a result of geographical distance. Geographical proximity, together with gender, marital status and employment status of the grandparent and the age of the grandparent/grandchild have been shown to influence the extent and nature of intergenerational contact (Troll 1985; Johnson 1985; Cherlin and Furstenberg 1986).

The study

Both quantative and qualitative data were collected. First, a nationally representative telephone survey of 870 grandparents of all ages was carried out in 1999–2000 by the Office of National Statistics (ONS). An earlier kinship study also carried out by ONS was used as a sampling frame. Of the original 1167 grandparents identified, 1019 agreed to take part in a follow-up study and 870 interviews were achieved (753 by telephone and 117 face to face). This is a response rate of 75 per cent from the original sample and 86 per cent of those who agreed to be followed up. In contrast to most of the previous research which was focused on grandmothers, both men and women were invited to participate in the survey. The final sample included 521 women and 349 men.

The Omnibus Survey mapped numbers, ages and the family types of grandchildren, grandparental contact and grandparental attitudes to family relationships. Very importantly, its main advantage over previous British data is that it collected information about all sets of grandchildren; that is grandparents were asked about all sets of grandchildren defined as children living in the same household up to a maximum of five. Previous surveys have asked only about selected grandchildren due to the complexity of data collection for all grandchildren. It also collected information about attitudes to grandparenting and contact and quality of relationships.

Second, qualitative in-depth interviews with 45 grandparents were undertaken to investigate what meaning and value was attached to being a grandparent by older people and how this varied by their family circumstances and personal characteristics. Grandparents were selected from the Omnibus Survey for interview on the basis of their age, and the family type of their grandchildren; that is whether the parents were living together/married, separated /divorced and, where relevant, by whether they had grandchildren in intact and non intact families. Where possible the interview also included the partner of the primary respondent. In total 18 individual grandparents and 27 couples were interviewed. Using the age of the primary respondent, 13 of those interviewed were under 60 years of age, 18 were aged 60 to 69 and 16 were aged 70 and over.

We explored the extent to which current grandparenting roles and levels and types of activity are chosen by or constrained for older people and how this is related to their level of satisfaction with their experience of grandparenthood. We also wanted to establish the extent and nature of grandparents' financial, practical and emotional support for their children's families, and reasons for the variations in support and the reciprocal nature of this intergenerational exchange. Finally we explored the significance of older people's role as grandparents to both their identity as older people and to the emotional, social and financial quality of their lives. A key interest for us was the extent to which family break-up may have affected grandparents' role and activities.

A third stage was also undertaken when a two-month Omnibus Survey of 2011 grandparents in 2001 repeated the questions asked in the initial survey and asked further questions on the activities under-taken by grandparents. In this chapter we report briefly on the main findings from the national survey but the principal focus is on the in-depth accounts from grandparents of their experience of being a grandparent, its meaning and contribution to their quality of life.

Grandparents and their grandchildren

The grandparents showed great socio-demographic variability. The youngest grandparent interviewed was aged 37 years and the oldest was aged 94. These grandparents were not the stereotypical old and retired family member; one third were under 60 and another third between 60 and 69 years old, and many were in paid employment. The maximum number of grandchildren any grandparent had was 23 and the oldest grandchild was 52 years. The maximum number of sets (that is living together) of grandchildren was 20; this respondent was aged 82 and most of her grandchildren were older. It is likely that the majority of these children had left the family household, and as a consequence every individual represents a different set by our definition. The number of grandchildren and sets of grandchildren was related to socio-economic indicators, reflecting the higher birth rate amongst lower socio-economic groups, as well as the younger age at childbirth.

The quantitative survey confirmed our hypotheses that the families of the grandchildren were not uniform. Nearly one in four of grand-parents (38 per cent) had experienced family breakdown in at least one of their sets of grandchildren, and for 10 per cent this meant family breakdown in all sets of grandchildren. Family breakdown of grand-children's families was not related to socio-economic characteristics of the grandparent. Interestingly, over a fifth of grandparents interviewed had at least one step-grandchild and this was more common for grandparents who were younger than 70.

The effect of family change, particularly in more recent years (younger grandparents), is having a marked impact on grandparents as evidenced in the numbers of grandchildren and family patterns found in this study.

Contact with grandchildren has been cited as being crucially important for developing and maintaining a grandparent's relationship with grandchildren and popular debate suggests that a more geo-graphically mobile society has considerably reduced the opportunities for this (Dench and Ogg 2002). Here the powerful images of the 'nan round the corner' associated with the working-class communities which Townsend and Young and Willmott captured in their classic studies of Bethnal Green has shaped popular thinking. Clearly we would not expect a national study 50 years on and covering a much more diverse range of grandparents than these community studies encompassed to show the same close physical proximity. Yet by certain standards levels of contact seemed higher than expected. Table 10.1 shows that three in five grandparents saw at least one grandchild or set of grandchildren on a weekly basis and about the same proportion of grandparents (60 per cent) reported they had frequent contact by telephone, letter or email. Nearly two-thirds (64 per cent) of grandparents lived within half an hour of at least one grandchild and proximity was related to the age and social class of the grandparent: older grandparents and non-manual grandparents were less likely to see grandchildren on a weekly basis.

Table 10.1 Contact with grandchildren

	See grandchildren* %	Other contact** %
At least once a week	61	60
At least every month	17	12
Only in school holidays/ every three months	10	3
Less often	10	9
Never	2	16

* See any grandchild
** Telephone, letter, email, etc.

Contact was most closely related to the proximity of the grandparent to the grandchild. However, we do not know from this study whether residential decisions and housing moves were deliberately made to enable contact with grandchildren or children or whether contact happens because families were already in close proximity. As daughters are slightly more likely to live nearer their own parents than sons, whether by choice or 'accident' this is one factor which helps to make 'lineage' an important factor in predicting contact. Our analysis showed that lineage is more important to intensity of contact than whether or not the grandchildren are living in an intact family or not. Grandparents will see less of grandchildren through sons and a family break-up may exacerbate this. This confirms that family breakdown affects grandparent–grandchild contact and the relationship with the grandchildren's parents is particularly important when this occurs.

Meaning of grandparenthood and its contribution to quality of life of older people

Our study confirmed that family relationships today are complex and grandparenthood remains an important family relationship for older people in Britain. The survey revealed that 15 per cent of grandparents believed that their relationship with at least one set of grandchildren was 'the most important relationship' in their life and that 70 per cent thought it was 'one of the most important relationships' they had. Age did not significantly affect respondents' views on this. Ninety per cent of grandparents aged under 60 years old stated that the role was either 'the most important' or was 'one of the most important' relationships in their life and, similarly, this was true for 85 per cent of grandparents over 60 years old.

The marital status of the grandparent did have an effect on how important the relationship with grandchildren was perceived to be, although this was also affected by the gender of the respondent. Grandfathers appeared to be engaged in family networks and relationships by being married. Of the 340 grandfathers in our study, 84 per cent of those who were married or living with a partner said that their relationship with at least one set of their grandchildren was either the most important or one of the most important in their life. This compared with just 59 per cent of those grandfathers either not married or not living with a partner. There was no significant difference for grandmothers. This reflects the findings of Uhlenberg and Hammil (1998) which revealed that married grandfathers were twice as likely as widowed ones to see their grandchildren frequently and about half as likely to see them on an infrequent basis. Divorced, separated and remarried grandfathers were even less likely to have frequent contact with grandchildren.

The importance of the relationship with grandchildren also differed significantly by proximity, or how close they lived to grandchildren, and how often they saw them. Among grandparents who saw their grandchildren at least once a week, 18 per cent said that the relationship with at least one of their sets of grandchildren was the most important and 74 per cent said it was one of the most important relationships in their life. This compared with just 7 per cent and 65 per cent respectively of those who saw their grandchildren only in the school holidays. Grandparents who lived closer to their grandchildren also felt the relationship was more important to them. Among grandparents who lived within half an hour of at least one set of grandchildren, 17 per cent said that the relationship was the most important in their lives compared with just 11 per cent of those living within two hours and 6 per cent of those living more than two hours away. Overall the majority (55 per cent) of grandparents said that being a grandparent contributed 'enormously' to their quality of life and a third (31 per cent) said it contributed 'a lot'. Only 4 per cent felt it contributed 'not at all'.

The qualitative study also confirmed the importance of grandchildren to grandparents. Of the 45 grandparents interviewed in depth, 7 said that the grandparent–grandchild relationship was the most important in their life and 9 that it was an important relationship but not the central relationship in their lives. The majority of the grandparents stated that their relationship with grandchildren was one of the most important in their lives along with their relationships with their children and, if they had one, their partner.

We asked respondents what they felt contributed to or increased the quality of their lives. The primacy of family relations was paramount with relationships with family members, including children and grandchildren, mentioned the most often (28). Not surprisingly, for older people beginning to experience the worry or actuality of poorer health, 'good health' was the next most mentioned factor (13), followed by relationship with spouse or partner (9). Having sufficient money was mentioned eight times. Other factors believed to increase quality of life, in order of importance, were friends, being able to do things, work, holidays and being a member of a church/having faith. In contrast, the factors mentioned which undermined their quality of life were more tangible. Older people worried most about their own ill health or others (17) followed by financial worries (6), as well as work stress and not being mobile or able to get around. Family relationships did not figure as a detractor from a good quality of life for the vast majority of grandparents as it appeared the existence of these was taken for granted.

What was it about the grandparent–grandchild relationship which made it so special for most of the grandparents interviewed in this study? Cunningham-Burley's early work (1986) on the meaning of grandparenthood showed that for most grandparents grandparenthood is something that is very much taken for granted as a stage in life, part of the natural way of things. A grandchild personifies continuity within a lifetime as well as continuity across lifetimes, beyond death. Grandchildren are also seen as keeping grandparents young and providing new meaning to life.

The ONS survey findings revealed that although older grandparents did not see their grandchildren as often or participate in as many activities with their grandchildren, they rated the importance of the role as highly as did younger grandparents. So although contact and activities with grandchildren were investigated as the context of the operation of this relationship, it was also important to look at the meanings that the respondents themselves attached to the role irrespective of their behaviour. We began by asking grandparents about their feelings on becoming grandparents and then explored how becoming a grandparent impacted on their life in general, how they felt about this, what they felt the differences between parenthood and grandparenthood were and the perceived rewards and costs of grandparenthood.

Finding out about becoming a grandparent

Unlike parenthood, movement into this important stage of the life cycle is entirely out of the individual's control. One respondent talked about feeling shock at being told the news with the realisation that entry into grandparenthood is not something that you choose yourself, rather it is dependent upon the decisions of other people: 'You don't get a choice in the matter, you get told, you're informed, by the way ... yes pretty shocked I suppose.'

Many grandparents looked back on when they first became grandparents as a time of great happiness. Words such as 'delighted', 'thrilled', 'over the moon' were used to express this. To some becoming a grandparent was expected, it was something that was inevitable and even taken for granted. This was particularly the case where the parents had been married for a while: 'It was the natural order of things at the time because the parents had a stable marriage and it was very nice to look forward to and then see.'

Mixed feelings about becoming a grandparent were only expressed if the child was not in what was considered a suitable relationship or situation or if the child was moving into parenthood at what was considered a young age. In these circumstances happiness about becoming a grandparent was tempered by worry over the child and grandchild. Some respondents, however, did express personal reluctance, feeling they were too young to be making the transition to grandparenthood: 'Oh I'm too young. I did, I thought I'm only 43 and I'm too young to be a granny.' To these respondents movement into grandparenthood seemed to signify entry into old age. This initial reaction, however, soon gave way to joy at the birth of the child and further questioning revealed that grandchildren in fact made the grandparents feel younger rather than older.

The symbolic significance of grandparenthood

For many grandparents the transition to grandparenthood signified a sense of continuity and immortality. Great satisfaction was expressed that children had gone on to have their own children and thus the next generation was assured:

> [him] I suppose you've got the satisfaction of knowing that the generations are going to continue. I mean I've always felt sorry for families that couldn't or wouldn't have children or grandchildren.

> [her] It's sort of a feeling of they are ours and, sounds possessive that does doesn't it but you know what I mean ... they are our own blood, they are ours.

This sense of the family continuing was highly personal and great delight was taken in seeing family traits and characteristics being passed on: 'I think oh I wonder who he looks like you know, you see your own, well he's got my nails I know that and you know, has he got someone else's nose and eyes you know. It seems as though, well it's somebody what is taking after you, your family.'

Many of the grandparents felt that there would be something missing in life without grandchildren and that having them meant that something of themselves had been passed on to future generations. Linked to this was a feeling of investment and achievement, of having contributed to the development and personal growth of the grandchild. Many of the grandparents expressed a great sense of accomplishment and pride in their grandchildren and felt immense satisfaction in seeing them growing up to be well-rounded individuals: 'I always feel so much better when I've had the grandchildren round. I feel as if compared to work I've achieved something ... I've used my time usefully and you know they're kind of, if you like, the end product.'

For the majority of respondents the transition to grandparenthood symbolised a renewal of youth rather than movement into old age as one would expect. Grandchildren represented an increase in the pace of life, a return to activities that the grandparents remembered as parents: 'They keep you young don't they, you move up a step when your children grow up you slow down, settle into a sort of routine pattern. When they come along you have to move up about three notches, you have to go a lot faster.' Grandparenthood appeared to create links between the generations and symbolise the continuity of the generations and the family.

The difference between being a parent and being a grandparent

The one element of the grandparental role, which was mentioned by all grandparents, was that is was critically different from being a parent. Not only was it not in their control as to whether or when they became a grandparent, but there was a critical difference in terms of freedom from 'responsibility' for the children, which is the role of a parent. They expressed this as a liberating relationship; they were free to enjoy it without the responsibility for it. They also felt that they had greater freedom to discuss or express intimacies with older grandchildren which had been 'out of bounds' with their own children.

One respondent commented that it was 'the difference between a full-time and a part-time job'. The grandchildren are around for a limited amount of time, great fun is had and then they are handed back to their parents for the sleepless nights and the tantrums: 'It's like having a second go at it when you've got older really but you haven't got the responsibility have you, you've just got the pleasure.'

This certainly heightened the enjoyment of grandparenting for the respondents and many felt that they were more relaxed in their attitude compared to when they were parents. This was also supported by fewer concerns about money and being able to afford to bring up children. Many grandparents also reported having more time and patience for their grandchildren than they had for their own children and feeling more secure, capable and worldly wise and so better able to deal with young children than when they themselves were younger. As one grandmother said: 'When it's your grandchild it's different you know … there's not that sort of worry behind it and it's just a blessing you know … I think when you have a child, your own child, it's a mixed blessing whereas there's no mixed blessing about a grandchild.' Indeed many of the grandparents reported this lack of responsibility as the best thing about being a grandparent; getting all the perks and benefits of the children without the costs or burden.

At the same time, however, some of the grandparents felt that there was an increase in responsibility and worry – as one grandparent put it 'in some ways it's easier being a grandparent, in others it's not'. Grandchildren are additional members of the family and thus represent additional worry; they are 'something else that is yours to look after'. Other respondents reported being more afraid of something happening to the grandchildren while in their care than they had been about their own children: 'You haven't got that responsibility, but in another way if you take those two children on holiday you feel more responsible than if they were your own because you're accountable.'

Reorganising lives to include grandchildren – new activities and interests

Grandchildren were valued for the additional dimension they brought to grandparents' lives. Grandchildren 'keep you young … when they come along you have to move up a few notches … go a lot faster'. Becoming a grandparent signalled a major change in the lives of some older people. The addition of grandchildren to the family meant reorganising their time to fit in children, 'do what you want to do but now it's, you know, you have to sort of think'. The transition to grandparenthood refocused their lives to revolve around the family again, after concentrating more on themselves as individuals or a couple which had occurred when their own children left home. This was always a positive thing and as one couple stated: 'Otherwise you'd become too self-centred wouldn't you if it was just the two of you?'

Grandparenthood, for some respondents, meant that their lives became more busy or hectic. They took part in many more activities or some which they would not have done alone. Grandchildren meant altering routines for some of the grandparents. For others, although they did not have to change their lifestyle in any way, their grandchildren represented an additional point of interest in their lives: 'Well it gives you, well I suppose it's the extra interest. I mean when we see them we talk about what they're doing and school and what they're doing in sports ... it gives us something else to think about apart from ourselves doesn't it?' In this way grandchildren represented another element to the older people's lives, something that they could take part in, that extended what they themselves did and that provided a focus outside their own lives.

'You give a lot of love and you get a lot of love'

Many of the grandparents spoke of the unconditional love that grandchildren provide, particularly younger grandchildren. This was in fact one of the strongest themes to emerge from the interviews. One grandmother, for example, said: 'It's just the love that she gives back to you, you feel, well it just makes you feel complete somehow.' The grandchildren, again particularly the younger grandchildren, were quoted as being very vocal and demonstrative about their love for their grandparents and many of the respondents reported how happy it made them feel when their grandchildren hugged them, told them how much they loved them or simply drew pictures for them. As one grandparent said: 'It's those kinds of things that are really special, that's what it's all about isn't it?' Many people also talked about the sheer pleasure gained just from seeing the grandchildren and knowing that their pleasure is mirrored by their grandchildren's delight at seeing them. Linked to this is the feeling of being cared about and wanted just for who you are: 'Well it's the fact that you're wanted so much as you get older, you feel somebody really wants you, they like us ... I think that's what it's about.'

The relationship with grandchildren added to quality of life for many people just because it was a relationship based on a love that was unconditional and accepting. One grandparent expressed this by saying:

'I mean they don't get paid for anything ... it's nice to feel that they're pleased with whatever you do genuinely. It's not an artificial thing which is rewarding in itself.'

Given previous reports of grandfathers being less involved in family networks we were surprised by how much grandfathers were involved in the lives of their grandchildren. Many reported being actively engaged with grandchildren and also spoke of their attachment and love for grandchildren. There were poignant examples of grandfathers taking on an active male role when families had separated and feeling responsible for giving children the experience of being in a 'couple' family.

'It keeps us involved, gives us things to do'

Many of the grandparents spoke of taking part in activities that they wouldn't otherwise do and this again kept them young. The exchange of ideas and conversation with grandchildren also had the same result. In fact some older people felt that their lives would have been very different without grandchildren to give them this contact with youth: 'I'm sure they keep you young, cause if you didn't have young grandchildren around you, running around and keeping you young, you'd probably sit there and fade away or something.' As noted earlier, it also meant taking part in activities with their grandchildren that they thoroughly enjoyed but would never dream of doing on their own.

Seeing grandchildren and finding things to do with them gave older people something to look forward to and many found the time spent with their grandchildren fulfilling. Many grandparents reported feeling younger because of this relationship, 'it's an excuse to go back to your childhood'. They felt that grandchildren gave them the incentive to get up and do things they wouldn't normally do, to experience more in life whilst learning at the same time and life had become more hectic as a result: 'It's fun isn't it, sort of gets you out of a rut if you haven't got a lot planned for the weekend you've got something to do.'

For those grandparents who were unable to have an active role in their grandchildren's lives, for example, if they suffered from ill health or simply lived too far away, this contact and interest in their grand-children's lives still remained. Their rooms were filled with pictures of grandchildren and they were a major point of conversation.

'It's the joy of sharing with them'

Many older people gained great pleasure just from seeing their grandchildren happy, felt pride in their achievements and even felt it was important to participate in both the good and bad times of their lives: 'It gives you pleasure to see if they're happy and you're upset if they're upset, or at least that's how I find it.' They gained great satisfaction from seeing the grandchildren pleased, particularly if it was with something that they themselves had done. For some of the grandparents being able to contribute to their grandchildren's lives, helping out with money or simply buying gifts, gave great pleasure,

Many of the grandparents experienced a feeling of investment and achievement, of being able to contribute to the development and personal growth of the grandchild: 'I should say it's rewarding in that you know you can help and hopefully help to bring him up to be a decent citizen.' There was a sense of great pride if the grandchildren accomplished something in life. As one grandparent said: 'When they do achieve then you achieve in some way.' Many of the grandparents also mentioned gaining happiness through their own children benefiting from becoming parents.

'I think it would be very lonely without them'

For some people becoming a grandparent increased their contact with both family members and other people within the community. Grandchildren also assured continuity within the family and, in many instances, meant increased contact with children. Some grandparents mentioned feeling closer to the family generally after grandchildren were born. One reason for this was felt to be that their children had 'settled down', decided to become a parent and to a certain extent changed in their outlook: 'It's different once they've got children because they change and they, their interests are different and they become more like yours perhaps.'

More involvement with other members of the community was also a facet of grandparenthood for a few people. In particular, one grandmother who took her granddaughter to nursery group said: 'It's nice to be involved like all the young mums, it's lovely actually that side of it, you know you're treated the same as you were when they were your children, yes that's what I think is rather nice.' Another couple felt that they had become linked to the wider local community through their grandchildren. They reported getting to know other people in the neighbourhood with children, some of whom had become friends. As the grandmother said: 'It's like another life, it's strange actually.'

Can grandparenthood detract from quality of life?

A small number of grandparents reported negative elements involved in being a grandparent. In all cases these people were doing more or different things than they had anticipated doing as grandparents. In one extreme case a grandfather was acting as a parent in the absence of his daughter and had taken on this role rather than see his grand-daughter adopted. This certainly had a major impact on his life which, taken overall, was disruptive and not beneficial. When asked how his life had changed he said:

> I don't want to use the word burden but yeah it's changed my life and not for the better ... If I hadn't stepped in and done this she would have been adopted and I wouldn't have seen her and that's why I stepped in and took custody. It wasn't ideal but then again I want to see my granddaughter so in a way I wouldn't say I've ruined my life but I've basically put, it's like putting your life on hold you know for what is going to be ten, fifteen years, I don't know.

The situation had forced this respondent to step out of the grand-parental into a parental role with full responsibility for his granddaughter at a time perhaps when he was looking forward to living his own life. As a result the respondent did not feel that he was a 'normal' grandparent.

Other people who expressed some adverse effects of grand-parenthood said this was because they were asked to do too much or because it was taken for granted that they would help. This theme of overburden was particularly related to childcare. Some grandparents felt they had to help daughters or daughters-in-law, who were struggling to manage children and paid work, without access to affordable or suitable childcare or in families which rejected non-family care for young children. These expectations were clearly resented but seen as a 'Hobson's choice' and these grandparents clearly felt it was better for them to be inconvenienced than either their children give up work or their grandchildren have care which the family deemed inappropriate.

This group of grandparents differed importantly from the small minority of grandparents who felt they were 'put upon' by unthinking or selfish children who expected them to do a lot of childcare or babysitting with little appreciation. This thoughtlessness could distress grandparents, though some reported that they sometimes resisted the pressures by setting firm boundaries. As one said: 'I've told them to count me out unless they are in real trouble, then I will. I'll be here but I am not a built in babysitter, I've got my own life and they all understand that.'

Conclusions

Family relationships are more complex today than in previous eras but grandparenthood remains an important family relationship for older people in Britain. There is great variation between grandparents, however, in how this role operates. There is evidence too that family change is affecting the grandparent role. One in four grandparents had grandchildren living in separated families and one in five had step-grandchildren. However, despite this, grandparents were unanimous in reporting that grandparenthood was an important part of their life and most felt it contributed 'enormously' to their quality of life.

The importance of this family role for older people was partly reflected in the frequency with which many grandparents saw grand-children; six out of ten grandparents saw at least one grandchild or set of grandchildren once a week. The same proportion of grandparents reported other contact via telephone, letter or email. Weekly contact was related most strongly to proximity (how close they lived) but lineage (whether through sons or daughters) was more important than family type. Grandparents were less likely to see grandchildren through sons on a weekly basis, especially if they had experienced family break-up, than those through daughters.

When the meaning of grandparenthood for older people was explored it was clear that this role was not chosen by the grandparent but was a consequence of the decisions and actions of others and the timing may not be something older people would chose. But for the vast majority of grandparents it was a role they welcomed and enjoyed. The relationship between grandparent and grandchild was char-acterised in the minds of most grandparents by a sense of strong emotional closeness and many grandparents experienced having grandchildren as very rewarding. They were alive to the marked difference in being a grandparent compared with a parent and enjoyed the 'part-time' nature of the position and the ability to 'hand them back'.

There was too an important symbolic value of grandchildren. They represented a sense of continuity and immortality – the family carrying on – and linked to this was a sense of achievement: – 'I feel as if compared to work I've achieved something ... I've used my time usefully and they are kind of like the end product.' But equally grandchildren were valued for the additional dimension they brought to grandparents' lives. Grandparents reported doing things they wouldn't otherwise have done and felt these new experiences kept them young and involved in the world. Contrary to previous reports, we found that grandfathers were often closely involved in the lives of their grandchildren. Many reported being actively engaged with grandchildren and also spoke of their attachment and love for grandchildren.

Finally, respondents' reactions to first becoming grandparents reflected the stereotypical picture of grandparents still held in the wider population. Many said they felt 'odd' when they first knew they were to become a grandparent as they did not think of themselves as a typical grandparent, which they defined as an elderly, often ill, 'distant' or 'removed' grandparent not engaged in a practical way with grandchildren. This was at odds with both how these grandparents wanted to be and their experiences as grandparents.

11

Frailty and institutional life

Susan Tester, Gill Hubbard, Murna Downs, Charlotte MacDonald and Joan Murphy

Introduction

This research focuses on the quality of life of frail older people living in institutional care. We defined frail older people as those with severe physical and/or mental conditions or disabilities during the period at the end of their lives. This 'fourth age' is often perceived negatively (Featherstone and Hepworth 1993; Bytheway 1995). The current policy emphasis on the third age may further marginalise and stigmatise the oldest and frailest groups, particularly when they are in institutional care. In the context of such negative attitudes in wider society, our research set out to examine the quality of life of frail older people in care homes and identify ways in which they could experience a good quality of life. In particular the main aim of the research was to contribute to understanding the meaning of quality of life for frail older people from the perspectives of older people themselves.

The study explored quality of life within the context of the transition to institutional care by eliciting perceptions of quality of life of frail older people who had moved into care homes in the six months prior to participation in the research. Research on the effects of transition to institutional care on quality of life is equivocal. Lieberman (1991), for example, has drawn attention to the need to form new attachments and the need for psychological work in adapting to a major life change, but found no direct answers to explain the effects of relocation. Oldman and Quilgars (1999) found that in some ways the move into residential care could be perceived positively. Reberger et al. (1999) found that older people who moved into hostel care reported an improvement in their physical, cognitive and social functioning, but not in their mental health. Continuities and discontinuities with life before the move may have positive or negative impacts and residents develop personal strategies for adaptation to the new environment (Reed and Roskell Payton 1996).

Of course quality of care can contribute to quality of life in the care home and much previous research has stressed the negative aspects of care and of life in residential and nursing care homes (Peace et al. 1997). Since the 1980s, policy emphasis on quality assurance and outcomes of care has promoted qualitative models for evaluating quality of life in care homes, using the basic values of privacy, dignity, independence, choice, rights and fulfilment, and drawing on the subjective experiences of residents and staff (DoH/SSI 1989; Kellaher 1998). National care standards have been introduced in England and Wales (DoH 2003) under the Care Standards Act 2000; and in Scotland (Scottish Executive 2001) under the Regulation of Care (Scotland) Act 2001. These care standards are integral to new systems of inspection and regulation of care that take account of residents' perspectives on quality of life.

Methodology and methods

Quality of life has rarely been studied from the perspectives of frail older people. Those with the most severe disabilities and with whom communication is difficult are often excluded from research (Farquhar 1995). Most quality of life studies of older people have been quantitative (Arnold 1991). Our research took a subjective qualitative approach to quality of life starting from the view that 'quality of life is a dynamic interaction between the external conditions of an individual's life and the internal perceptions of those conditions' (Browne et al. 1994: 235). This approach assumes that feelings and judgements about life are 'intrinsic, subjective matters' (Farquhar 1995: 1440) and that an individual's perception of good quality of life is embedded within the context of personal values, goals, talents, histories, and life experiences (Faden and German 1994: 542).

Our central focus on understanding the meaning of quality of life for frail older people from their own perspectives therefore posed methodological challenges and required developing innovative methods of eliciting participants' views on this topic. Because we aimed to include people with all types of physical and/or mental disabilities or conditions an ethnographic approach (Hammersley and Atkinson 1995) using a range of qualitative observational and interview methods was employed. In exploring quality of life we used an interactionist approach to understand the symbolic worlds and shared meanings of frail older residents and the ways in which they negotiated meanings through their social interaction (Blumer 1969).

The research fieldwork was carried out in three stages, primarily in two health board areas of Scotland. In order to identify the quality of life issues most salient to older people themselves, the fieldwork began with six focus groups in the community, with older people and carers who were not yet frail. In Scotland we included a group of frail older people, family carers of older people with dementia, and women belonging to a friendship club. In Bradford (England) we held discussions with Asian men's and women's groups (Hubbard et al. 2001). Drawing on the qualitative methods of a pilot study (Hubbard et al. 2002) and using a framework based on the literature and focus group findings, the second stage involved naturalistic observation undertaken by the research team in four care home settings in Scotland. In each setting, observation was carried out in periods of two hours at a time during the day and a longer period at night, covering each day of the week and over 24 hours. The third stage used guided conversations and individual observation with a sample of 52 residents selected from seven care homes (six nursing homes and one residential care home) in Scotland. The participants included 41 women and 11 men, with ages ranging from the 65 to 69 age group to 95 to 99; the majority were in the 75 to 89 age range. In one home which catered for Jewish people, five residents were interviewed and in another home three Chinese residents were interviewed by a Chinese-speaking interviewer. We had aimed to include other groups but found that no residents from other minority ethnic groups had recently moved into the homes.

We elicited the views of each of the 52 participants through their verbal and non-verbal responses during two or more sessions. The first session with each individual began with observation. This was used to identify one of three strategies for the next session:

- a guided conversation with an interviewer

- a guided conversation using *Talking Mats*®, a visual framework that uses picture symbols to help people with a communication difficulty

- a series of shorter individual observation and intermittent conversation sessions with people with severe cognitive difficulties (Hubbard et al. 2003c).

Ten interviews were completed using *Talking Mats*® (Murphy 2003).

A rigorous approach was taken to data analysis in which the data were scrutinised continuously throughout the fieldwork and analysis stages, using an iterative process (Hammersley and Atkinson 1995:205). Field notes and transcripts were coded using frameworks developed and built upon as each stage progressed and the qualitative data software package NUD*IST 4 was used to facilitate analysis. Video recordings, field notes and digital photographs of completed mats from interviews using *Talking Mats*® were analysed using cognitive mapping (Jones 1985) and subsequently incorporated into the findings of the wider study.

Key findings

In exploring quality of life among the study participants we identified four key interrelated areas which they perceived to be the main components of quality of life: sense of self, the care environment, relationships, and activities. Having the opportunity to 'be oneself' in these ways was critical to quality of life and we examine each of them below. In analysing the findings we explored what 'sense of self' meant in the context of a care home, and the extent to which people were supported in 'being themselves'.

The transition to institutional care for people with developing frailties can entail threats to the person's self, autonomy and relationships (Bruce et al. 2002; Goffman 1961; Kitwood 1997). In exploring ways in which participants were able to be themselves after the transition to the care home, we found that they experienced different degrees of continuity or discontinuity with sense of self, autonomy and relationships. Such continuities and discontinuities could reduce or enhance quality of life, depending on the individual concerned. Participants developed different strategies for adapting to life in a care home, for example, distancing themselves from others seen as 'different', or adapting their environment to suit themselves.

A variety of factors influenced quality of life in positive or negative ways. These included the person's frailty and strength, gender, social class and ethnicity. The broader cultural and structural contexts and spiritual environments of the care homes and their residents also influenced frail older people's reported quality of life. Cultural facets of context included the local culture of the group of residents and the culture of care operating within specific homes. Structural facets of context were framed by resources, staffing and distribution of public and private space (Gubrium 1995; Hubbard et al. 2003c: 109–10). Communication was a key factor in quality of life. For frail older people to be able to express themselves, maintain a sense of self, form and maintain relationships, participate in interaction and activities and make meaning of their experiences it was essential to be able or enabled to communicate verbally and non-verbally.

Sense of self

The 52 study participants had a range of combinations of physical and mental conditions and disabilities; 24 of them had a diagnosed dementia. The meanings made by participants of their own and others' frailties and the responses of other residents, care staff, relatives and visitors had an impact on their quality of life. Focus group participants stressed the importance of recognising individuals' strengths, pointing out that older people are never 'really frail' as they can assert themselves in various ways to compensate for their frailty. We found, as did Kellaher (2000), that residents were able to maintain a sense of self in their new surroundings and that there were various means by which they were enabled or inhibited in doing so.

Many participants in care homes were ambivalent about their situation, not wanting to acknowledge their dependence but at the same time being resigned to it. People's degree of resignation about being frail and dependent on others was related to their loss of health and fitness rather than their chronological age. Perceptions about frailty were generally expressed relatively, referring to other residents in the homes. While many people expressed resignation to their frailty, some occasionally showed anger at their situation.

People expressed their identity through their appearance and this presentation of self was part of adaptation to life in a home. Women spoke more about their appearance and dress than did men and it was clear that being able to wear and look after clothes that they liked was an important source of self-respect and continuity with the rest of their lives. The impact of the transition to the home was evident in the view that some clothes or jewellery were 'too good' to be worn there and the suggestion that they had reached a stage of life where such accoutrements were inappropriate. The way the home provided help with getting dressed, shaving, hairdressing and nail varnishing was seen as adding to or detracting from how good people felt about themselves.

In many cases there were few personal possessions on show. The amount of personal storage space and concerns about security might affect what possessions people had brought with them from home. However, there was also some evidence that people felt that they no longer needed many possessions. In some cases there was undoubtedly a conscious choice not to adopt the home as a substitute for their own home by personalising their environment, but to maintain a sense of home as being their own house and possessions to which they might at some time return. There was no noticeable difference in the attachment to possessions expressed by men and women.

Lack of privacy in care homes was an issue raised by the focus groups and the interviews showed that it was clearly important for residents to be offered a choice of different levels of privacy. Peace and quiet was a high priority for some who valued the opportunity to keep themselves apart from the crowd. Others liked to be among other people whether or not they were actually socialising; something that they may have missed while living at home. The frailer residents had less control over where they spent their time than less frail residents as they were dependent on care staff to assist them in moving.

Participants in care homes thus expressed their sense of self through meanings made of and responses to their own and others' frailties and strengths, and through their personal appearance and possessions and preferences for personal space. People's ability to feel 'at home' in the home was reflected in how they dressed, items they chose to bring into the home and control over personal space. Their quality of life was inhibited if they were unable to feel 'at home' in the home and to feel comfortable in expressing their sense of self positively. This inability to feel 'at home' was expressed in frequent references to going home, only staying a short time, and not accepting being in the home. Some participants perceived the home as a place where they were waiting to die rather than as a place to live. It was clearly important for other residents, care staff and visitors to support participants in expressing their sense of self, being able to feel at home and enjoying positive quality of life in the care environment.

The care environment

To maintain a sense of self it is essential for people to have some control over daily living. We explore below the ways in which our participants lost control and were controlled in the care home environment but also ways in which they asserted or were enabled to assert control, choices or rights. In many cases lack of autonomy was attributed to physical and mental limitations, but the environment and care regime of the home also restricted residents' agency. The home environment, including the physical layout of the building, provided the structural context in which participants experienced their daily lives, whereas the care they received was influenced by the local culture of the home (Gubrium 1995).

Participants' reactions to the home environment and the care they received were expressed in positive terms as having choices and opportunities to do things which allowed residents to 'be themselves', and in negative terms as restrictions which limited residents' activities or led to uneasiness or discomfort. Having choices, expressing preferences and opinions and making complaints were all ways in which participants might express themselves as individuals. Finding fault with aspects of home life and talking about making complaints was revealing of self-respect and a sense of autonomy, in spite of the institutional setting.

In general people accepted or tolerated the care homes' rules and timetables. However, some participants were angry or frustrated by a loss of freedom expressed in terms of feeling controlled or under surveillance. Others valued opportunities to be independent and there was some evidence of people making a conscious effort to adapt the environment to suit themselves. Although staff controlled activities such as smoking, some residents asserted themselves by ignoring such controls.

Participants expressed positive and negative views on the effects of moving to a care home. Positive effects included being looked after and having cooking, cleaning and washing done by others, a discontinuity that enhanced quality of life through delegated agency; whereas negative effects included loss of freedom of movement. The findings showed that since many residents required help with mobility and self-care, carers could control their movement and the amount of self-care accomplished by residents. Some carers were able to support residents' agency by interpreting their non-verbal behaviour as signs that they wanted to take control.

Compatibility of pace between residents and staff was important (Kitwood 1997). Staff did not spend much time in assisting mobility except when it was necessary for mealtimes, getting up and going to bed and visits to the toilet. However, people were remarkably accepting of this. There was less tolerance about not being able to get to the toilet when necessary. Perhaps the most fundamental aspect of agency is evident in our control over going to the toilet. People described the embarrassment, discomfort and indignity of having accidents, being left too long on the toilet or having to wear incontinence pads. Side-effects of medication were seen as part of the trouble but there was evidence of incontinence pads being used for people who had bladder control but lacked mobility.

Being able to express preferences for food was an important way of maintaining a sense of self. Some people clearly appreciated being catered for and being offered food they liked. A few unfavourable comments suggested that low-cost convenience food was used rather than the kind of wholesome food which they enjoyed. Other comments about not enough being provided for breakfast suggested that the homes' priorities were not always seen by residents as matching their own.

Good quality of life was promoted by staff paying attention to personal needs in a caring way. Criticisms of personal care expressed by participants stemmed from inadequate staff time for individual care and lack of respect for individuals. Small details in the care relationship could have a major impact on an individual's quality of life (Bruce et al. 2002). The characteristics and approach of individual members of staff varied and could enhance quality of life through personal relationships and friendliness, or inhibit it through rough handling and lack of respect in manner or speech.

Relationships

A fundamental aspect of 'being oneself' is the ability to form and maintain personal relationships. Older people living at home, alone or with a spouse and who have limiting illnesses are likely to have reduced social networks and less social contact than others. Therefore, moving into a home could provide an opportunity to overcome social isolation and improve quality of life through social interaction and new relationships. On the other hand, people moving into homes may become cut off from past associations with neighbours, friends and family, particularly if the home is not close to where they used to live. For some of our participants loss of familiar company was experienced as a negative effect of moving to the home. We explore below ways in which participants were able to maintain a sense of self through relationships with others in the home and with family members and others outside the home.

The findings show that participants did have a sense of self in relation to others and were able to take on the role of others to interpret behaviour, make meaning of it and react to it (Hubbard et al. 2002: 159). The presence of others who were mentally frail was used to give people a point of comparison for their own mental state (Goffman 1968). Some residents reacted to others' behaviour with hostility. They labelled others as 'mental' or 'funny types' and distanced themselves from these roles; for example, by colonising particular lounges to avoid those labelled as 'mental', thus projecting their 'self' as 'not mental' (Hubbard et al. 2003c: 108–11). For people with dementia their disorientation seemed to make it harder to be understood by other residents and the disorientation of others may have added to their own.

Within care homes, verbal and non-verbal communication and meaningful social interaction are crucial for sense of self, for development and maintenance of relationships with other residents and for quality of life. However, communication and interaction are often impeded by speech and hearing impairments (Kovach and Robinson 1996). Practical barriers such as loss or non-use of hearing aids unnecessarily affected communication. Non-verbal communication by those with sensory and/or cognitive impairments conveys feelings and meanings, and allows for participation in social interaction and the development of relationships (Hubbard et al. 2002: 164).

Although lack of social interaction has often been emphasised, particularly in quantitative research on institutional care – the 'hours of nothingness' described by one focus group – our findings show that communication and social interaction did take place. Examples included talking, miming, using humour, jokes and teasing (Hubbard et al. 2003c). The findings revealed a range of feelings and emotions about other residents, as one would expect in any group of people living together. Attitudes towards other residents included hostility and indifference as well as sympathy and friendship. It was not uncommon for other residents to be portrayed as irrelevant to or only detracting from quality of life. Men tended to express this more openly than women but the underlying sense was similar.

Much of the interaction between residents seemed to arise from proximity rather than choice, similar to interaction between strangers. Group activities such as meals and recreation triggered interaction of a more sociable kind, but did not necessarily suit all tastes. In spite of the barriers, friendship and friendliness towards other residents was evident, although having a particular friend among the residents seemed to be a rare and valuable asset. Some connection from the past or a shared experience had provided the basis for friendship.

Participants also had sexual selves, as seen in the general observation in homes. They expressed their sexuality through their dress and appearance, in humorous discussions (particularly between women) about sexual relationships, and in flirting and displays of affection between men and women, including romantic and sexual affection, particularly in one care home (Hubbard et al. 2003c; Hubbard et al. 2003a). Some of the interview participants discussed sexual relationships, or lack of opportunity for them, particularly for women since there were few male residents.

Older people consider family relationships and social contacts as valuable for quality of life (Farquhar 1995). Among our participants, whether or not the husband or wife was still alive, married life contributed a great deal to quality of life, providing a store of memories and a sense of identity. In exceptional cases, the level of involvement of spouses or other close family members seemed high enough to affirm the resident's sense of being an active member of their family. It seemed from our analysis that the level of involvement of relatives in their lives could make a perceptible difference to people's self-confidence and their ability to relate to the home and the people in it.

For people with dementia, relationships with spouses, parents and siblings who may no longer be alive seemed salient to their present quality of life. Opportunities to talk about family memories from the past appeared important. As Mills and Coleman (1994) show, although cognitive functioning is in decline, people with dementia can recall parts of their past biographies. Older people with dementia can be supported in retaining a sense of self by encouraging them to talk about their life history, building on the strengths of emotional memories of the self (Mills 1997).

Our analysis also pointed to changes in relationships with children who might have been instrumental in arranging the move to the home and who might assume more authority in their parents' lives than in the past. The care and concern of relatives was evidenced in regular and frequent visiting and also in gifts and services performed. This undoubtedly added to the resident's sense of self-worth. Lack of involvement on the part of children was a cause for discontent in some cases, though some were more open in their criticism than others. Visitors, whether or not they were close relatives, clearly had great potential as sources of interest and social stimulation for groups of residents as well as for individuals.

Activities

In talking about how they spent their time in the home, people revealed more about themselves and their interests and how these had carried over or changed from their previous life. In some cases we have evidence of what people liked doing but were not able to do now that they lived in the home. Everyday activities such as getting up, having meals and cups of tea and going to bed provided the main activities of the day and these followed a routine for most residents. For some people this seemed to be as much as they wanted to cope with, while others were clearly bored and frustrated. Women seemed more inclined to express this kind of negative feeling in the interviews than men. In between the routine activities, the time was spent sitting in armchairs and many different modes of involvement and lack of involvement were experienced at these times.

Some found stimulation and pleasure in the kind of activities which they would have enjoyed in their own homes: watching the view from a window, or engaging in hobbies such as reading, sewing and listening to music. Others admitted that they had given up these kinds of pastimes and there often seemed to be a dearth of stimulation for them. The general observation provided some evidence of staff engaging in specific activities with residents or giving personal attention designed to stimulate or entertain people. In some cases spiritual needs were met through taking part in religious observance which was important for some participants in and of itself or as an enjoyable activity involving singing and music.

Getting out of the home was a fairly rare occurrence. Regular visits to family homes were very important for those who had families nearby. Other kinds of outings were rarely referred to except as something that participants would like rather than as something that actually happened. Having relatives to arrange such outings was usually welcome although anxiety about getting to the toilet could spoil the enjoyment. For most residents the lack of opportunity to go out meant that it was no longer possible to be involved in the local community or enjoy such activities as going window shopping or having a pint in the pub.

Although weekly bingo and dominoes sessions were referred to in other homes, only one of those studied had daily recreational activities organised. Organised activities were obviously enjoyable to those who took part, many of whom had dementia (Hubbard et al. 2003b: 357). These activities were sociable and also gave people a sense of achievement from learning to play the games. The activities that were provided did not suit all tastes and some participants stressed that it was important to be able to opt out as well as to participate.

Quality of life of frail older people

Despite the negative perceptions of and attitudes to frail older age and to life in care homes, we were able to observe and elicit some perceptions of good quality of life which allowed frail older people to 'be themselves'. Examples include asserting control, enjoyment of small pleasures such as the view from the window, 'pockets of interaction', humour, being part of a family and having a friend.

Participants' perceptions and experiences were also affected by their gender, social class and ethnicity. There were differences between men and women in the salience of appearance, as women were more likely than men to express individuality and interest in their appearance and more likely to form friendly relationships. There were differences in how men and women spent their time. The Chinese participants' lives seemed to have some distinctive qualities based on shared cultural interests. In the Jewish home residents experienced specific features based on their cultural and religious backgrounds. In some cases there was evidence that feeling different from other residents because of social class background had an impact on quality of life. However, the personal, cultural and structural facets of context in which frail older people with different intersections of gender, class and ethnicity experienced their lives in care homes also had key impacts on the individual's quality of life and inequalities in quality of life between frail older people.

Quality of life was thus influenced in positive or negative ways. The key positive impacts on quality of life were the older person's strengths in response to frailty; being able to assert control and rights; validation of the person's emotional needs; experiencing meaningful communication and being able or enabled to communicate; gains and positive continuities from transition to the care home; advantages from gender, social class and ethnicity; a supportive spiritual environment; and positive cultural and structural contexts. Key negative impacts on quality of life were negative responses to the person's frailty and dependence; loss of control and being controlled; neglecting the person's emotional needs and experience; lack of meaningful communication and/or communication difficulties; losses and negative discontinuities from transition to the care home; disadvantages from gender, social class and ethnicity; failure to support the person's spiritual needs; and negative cultural and structural contexts.

Our framework for understanding quality of life in frail older age within institutional care, recognising the diversity of frail older people and giving central place to the frail older individual, is summarised in Figure 11.1.

Main implications for policy and practice

Conceptualisation of quality of life in frail older age has been primarily negative and based on the perceptions of people who are not old and frail.

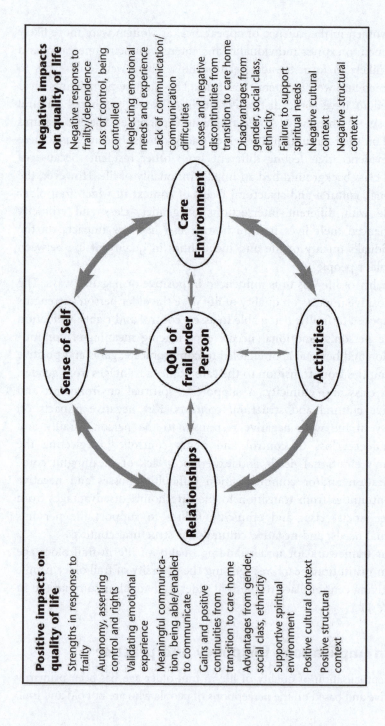

Positive impacts on quality of life

Strengths in response to frailty

Autonomy, asserting control and rights

Validating emotional experience

Meaningful communication, being able/enabled to communicate

Gains and positive continuities from transition to care home

Advantages from gender, social class, ethnicity

Supportive spiritual environment

Positive cultural context

Positive structural context

Negative impacts on quality of life

Negative response to frailty/dependence

Loss of control, being controlled

Neglecting emotional needs and experience

Lack of communication/ communication difficulties

Losses and negative discontinuities from transition to care home

Disadvantages from gender, social class, ethnicity

Failure to support spiritual needs

Negative cultural context

Negative structural context

Care Environment

Sense of Self

QOL of frail order Person

Activities

Relationships

Figure 11.1 Framework for understanding quality of life of frail older people in care homes

The contexts and contents of frail older people's lives are different from those of younger people. The assumptions made by policymakers, service providers and practitioners about what is important to frail older people in care homes may not be relevant. Thus, to promote quality of life in frail older age it is important that policymakers, service providers and professionals disregard their own assumptions and focus on the different priorities held by frail older people. This entails allowing or enabling frail older people to express their own preferences.

Our research developed successful innovative methods of eliciting frail older people's views and perceptions of quality of life across all types of physical and/or mental frailty. *Talking Mats*™ proved an effective method of gaining views that a frail older person may not otherwise be able to communicate and, in particular, helped people to express their feelings about different activities, showing clear likes and dislikes. The method can easily be used by professional or family carers to get to know the person, hold a conversation, elicit views on preferences for care or activities, or explore sensitive issues (Murphy 2003). Enabling people with severe communication difficulties to express their views and choices can in itself enhance quality of life. The importance of non-verbal communication of emotional expression as well as verbal communication must be recognised (Hubbard et al. 2002).

Our research found that it was possible to elicit their perceptions of quality of life from people with dementia using different methods tailored to the individual person. We also found that individual interviews and observation were 'meaning-making occasions'. Observation was helpful in meaning-making about the present and interviews in meaning-making about the past. Both methods can be used by carers in meaning-making in care homes (Hubbard et al. 2003b: 360).

Key principles for good practice with frail older people have been developed and widely accepted. These have recently been incorporated in new systems and care standards implemented in the UK. However, we found evidence of poor practice as well as good practice. The opportunities were limited for professional carers to support older people to be themselves, develop relationships and have meaningful interaction. In order to provide high quality care, staff need to have time to know and understand the individual.

In summary, quality of life can be promoted by good quality individualised care. This study demonstrates the key role that care providers and practitioners can play in enabling residents to maintain their sense of self, to communicate verbally and non-verbally, to exercise control and rights, to maintain and develop relationships, and to have meaningful activity and interaction within the contexts of institutional care settings.

Acknowledgements

The project (L480254023) formed part of the ESRC Growing Older Programme. The research team would like to acknowledge the specific contributions of Ailsa Cook, to papers based on this project and her ESRC PhD research, Mike Wilson for coding of data into NUD*IST and Sherry Macintosh for conducting the interviews with Chinese participants. We are grateful to all the participants, staff and managers of the homes included in the study. We also gratefully acknowledge the advice and contributions of the project advisory group, colleagues, research postgraduates and GO Programme participants.

12

Conclusion

Catherine Hagan Hennessy

It is not necessary to summarise the contents of the book as Chapter 1 provided an overview and each of the projects reported in Chapters 2 to 11 has produced a summary 'Findings' document (available on the GO Programme website – www.shef.ac.uk/uni/projects/gop/). It is worth mentioning in passing though that there are several cross-cutting themes that run through these chapters and indeed the whole programme of 24 projects. These major parameters of the programme and of quality of life in old age are the meaning given to quality of life by older people, and the roles of the environment, participation and ethnicity. These and other key themes will be explored in the companion volume to this one which will be published later in the GO series.

The remainder of this brief concluding chapter is devoted to the future directions of UK research on the quality of life of older people and, specifically, to how interdisciplinary research can add to the massive fund of social science evidence compiled by the GO Programme.

Future research on older people's quality of life

The Growing Older Programme has produced the largest systematic body of social science research regarding older people's quality of life to date in the UK. As demonstrated throughout this volume, this work has been far-ranging and has investigated many aspects of quality of life that have previously been neglected, wholly or partially. The output from the programme has included considerable new evidence regarding relationships between important social conditions and quality of life, which offer fresh support for the political economy of ageing paradigm (Chapter 1). The influence of structural factors such as social class, gender and ethnicity on quality of life in old age and over the life course is underscored heavily across the programme findings. In addition less well appreciated dimensions of and influences on quality of life, for example, existential concerns and individual agency among older people with cognitive impairments, were identified and examined in programme projects.

The richness of the programme findings reflects the innovativeness of the research designs and methods among the projects, including, for example, the use of large-scale, population-based survey data in conjunction with qualitative data from purposive samples drawn from the survey respondents (for example, in Chapters 2 and 3). In addition, the spectrum of phenomenologically oriented methods employed to achieve an understanding of older people's experiences of quality of life was impressive, ranging from individual in-depth qualitative interviews to focus groups, to novel techniques for eliciting the views of people with communication difficulties to the use of a participatory research approach. These methods also allowed for the greater inclusion of groups of older people whose views have been under-represented in quality of life research and for validation of measures and methods with these groups for whom the content validity of many existing quality of life scales has not been established (such as ethnic minority older people).

Findings from the Growing Older projects also suggest the way forward for research on older people's quality of life. The dynamic nature of the experience of loneliness described by Victor and her colleagues in Chapter 6, for example, and other project findings regarding social processes impinging on quality of life highlight the need for the use of longitudinal data in such investigations. The vast majority of the 24 programme projects, however, were based on cross-sectional data, with only two (Gilhooly et al.'s [2003] study of predictors of cognitive functioning and Blane et al.'s [2002] investigation of early and later life determinants of life satisfaction) employing over-time data. Given the growing importance of life course approaches to aspects of quality of life such as health which emphasise, for example, the cumulative effects of risk factors across the life span and the impact of resources acquired throughout life on the development of chronic diseases in old age (Kuh and Ben-Shlomo 1997), the need for longitudinal data is pressing. Likewise, definitive testing of theory-based hypotheses such as the experience of multiple jeopardy among ethnic minority older people examined in Nazroo et al.'s study (Chapter 3) will require longitudinal data (Markides and Black 1995). The mixed methods designs employed by many of the programme projects have been extremely fruitful in producing data on subjective as well as objective approaches to quality of life in old age. The continued use of quantitative and qualitative methods in longitudinal investigations would create a particularly powerful basis for researching quality of life processes and outcomes among older people.

The results of the programme projects also point to a role for the more explicit use of theory in future investigations of quality of life among older people. For example, many of the strategies employed by older people to accommodate to ageing related changes described in this volume can be systematically considered with reference to theoretical frameworks and related constructs from a variety of traditions, among them selective optimisation with compensation (Baltes and Carstensen 1999), the miniaturisation of satisfaction (Rubenstein et al. 1992), identity management, exchange theory (Marshall 1995) and gerotranscendence (Tornstam 1994). As research on quality of life progresses to increasingly make connections between macro-level social factors and processes and the micro-level experience of individuals, the utility of concepts and theories that can bridge these levels of analysis will become increasingly apparent (Marshall 1995). Likewise, the growing recognition of the value of interdisciplinary paradigms, models and methods in research on ageing that involves multiple levels of analysis, such as psychosocial and genetic determinants of health, will require greater cross-disciplinary collaboration by researchers (Kessel et al. 2003).

While the Growing Older Programme has significantly enhanced our understanding of the multiple dimensions of quality of life among older people and the range of factors contributing to it, only one of the 24 projects included in this portfolio examined a practical intervention related to quality of life – McKee et al.'s (2002) study of reminiscence. Numerous interventions, particularly those aimed at improving or maintaining the health status of older people, have produced a significant body of evidence regarding their impact on health-related quality of life. However, this research has been criticised as limited in its conceptualisation of quality of life outcomes by typically failing systematically to incorporate older people's views of appropriate outcomes, or to describe the contexts and processes involved in carrying out these interventions (Hennessy and Hennessy 1990). A significant role exists, therefore, for social scientists in intervention research related to older people's quality of life, including health and other dimensions of well-being. The importance of strategies for maintaining control and managing personal identity to quality of life documented throughout the programme findings would be of particular interest in regard to intervention research in this area.

A number of current developments in UK gerontological research offer substantial opportunities to address many of the research issues outlined above. Most significantly, the Economic and Social Research Council, which funded the Growing Older Programme, in partnership with the Medical Research Council, the Engineering and Physical Sciences Research Council and the Biotechnology and Biological Sciences Research Council, are funding a major new interdisciplinary programme of research on ageing to begin in 2004. The content of this programme was developed in consultation with the UK research community on ageing, including many of the Growing Older Programme researchers. Among the objectives of this programme, The New Dynamics of Ageing, are the exploration of lifecourse influences on individual ageing, and understanding the dynamic ways in which the meaning and experience of ageing are currently changing and becoming more diverse. The three substantive themes of the programme include areas that build on the Growing Older Programme findings: ageing well across the lifecourse, ageing and its environments, and innovative approaches to interdisciplinary research. Theoretically informed studies that examine interactions of factors relevant to quality of life over time and cross-sectionally and use innovative methodologies that span disciplines would make a valuable contribution to this research agenda.

This new programme on ageing is also informed by the National Collaboration on Ageing Research (NCAR) (www.sheffield.ac.uk/ukncar), a cross-Research Council partnership which was established in 2001 with the primary aim of stimulating interdisciplinary research in the field of ageing in the UK. The NCAR carries out a range of activities towards its twin objectives of building consensus among researchers and end users of research regarding priorities for interdisciplinary scientific collaboration and improving coordination among different research funders. These activities include conducting a series of topically based workshops which convene scientists from across the disciplines, as well as promoting the secondary use of existing UK data resources on ageing, including over 50 longitudinal datasets. The workshops have produced recommendations for cross-disciplinary research in a number of topic areas relevant to quality of life in older persons. These include, for example, health promotion and disability prevention, sensory impairments, influences on cognitive ageing and social and environmental supports for enhancing active ageing. The new cross-council ageing research programme offers ample scope for pursuing many of the interdisciplinary research agenda items which have emerged from the NCAR workshops and other activities. In addition, NCAR's work with a variety of stakeholders in ageing research, including policymakers, practitioners and older people themselves, will help to inform future research relevant to quality of life emerging from these interdisciplinary collaborations and in turn link resulting evidence to policy and practice.

Finally, echoing the introductory chapter, the Growing Older Programme set out to produce new scientific knowledge on older people's quality of life and the factors that contribute to it. As this volume has illustrated, the GO Programme has succeeded admirably in exploring quality of life in older age as a subjective, lived experience, as well as describing and identifying its context, variations and predictors among older people in the UK. These projects have also produced findings with significant implications for shaping the policies and practices that will ultimately enhance quality of life for current and future generations of older people.

Bibliography

6, P. (1997) Social exclusion: time to be optimistic, Demos Collection, 12:1–24.

Age Concern (1998) *Across the Generations*. London: Age Concern England.

Ahmad, W.I.U. (1996) Family obligations and social change among Asian communities, in W.I.U. Ahmad and K. Atkin (eds) *'Race' and Community Care*. Buckingham: Open University Press, pp. 51–72.

Ahmad, W.I.U. (2000) *Ethnicity, Disability and Chronic Illness*. Buckingham: Open University Press.

Ahmad, W.I.U. and Atkin, K. (1996) *'Race' and Community Care*. Buckingham: Open University Press.

Altman, I. and Low, S. (1992) *Place Attachment*. New York: Plenum Press.

Aldous, J. (1995) 'New views of grandparents in intergenerational context', *Journal of Family Issues*, 16(1): 104–22.

Andersson, L. (1998) Loneliness research and interventions: a review of the literature, *Ageing and Mental Health*, 2(4): 264–74.

Andrews, F.M. (ed.) (1986) *Research on the Quality of Life*. Michigan: Institute for Social Research, University of Michigan.

Andrews, F.M. and Withey, S.B. (1976) *Social Indicators of Well-being: Americans' Perceptions of Life Quality*. New York: Plenum Press.

Antonucci, T.C. and Akiyama, H. (1987) Gender and social support networks in later life, *Journal of Gerontology*, 42(5): 519–27.

Antonucci, T.C., Lansford, J.E., Schaberg, L. et al. (2001) Widowhood and illness: a comparison of social network characteristics in France, Germany, Japan, and the United States, *Psychology and Ageing*, 16(4): 655–65.

Arber, S. and Attias-Donfut, C. (eds.) (1999) *The Myth of Generational Conflict. The Family and State in Ageing Societies*. London: Routledge.

Arber, S. and Cooper, H. (1999) Gender differences in health in later life: the new paradox?, *Social Sciences and Medicine*, 48(1): 61–76.

Arber, S. and Ginn, J. (1991) *Gender and Later Life: A Sociological Analysis of Resources and Constraints*. London: Sage.

Arber, S. and Ginn, J. (eds) (1995) *Connecting Gender and Ageing: A Sociological Approach*. Buckingham: Open University Press.

Arnold, S. (1991) The measurement of quality of life in the frail elderly, in J. Birren, J. Lubben, J. Rowe and D. Deutchmann (eds) *The Concept and Measurement of Quality of Life in the Frail Elderly*. London: Academic Press.

Atkinson, R. and Davoudi, S. (2000) The concept of social exclusion in the European Union: context, development and possibilities, *Journal of Common Market Studies*, 38(3): 427–48.

Ayis, S., Gooberman-Hill, R. and Ebrahim, S. (2003) Long-standing and limiting illness in older people: associations with chronic diseases, psychosocial and environmental factors, *Age and Ageing*, 32(3): 265–72.

Bajekal, M., Blane, D., Grewal, I., Karlsen, S. and Nazroo, J. (2004) Ethnic differences in influences on quality of life at older ages: a quantitative analysis, *Ageing and Society*, in press.

Baltes, M.M. and Carstensen, L.L. (1999) Social-psychological theories and their applications to aging: from individual to collective, in V. Bengston and K. Schaie (eds) *Handbook of Theories of Aging*. New York: Springer, pp. 209–26.

Baltes, P.B. and Baltes, M.M. (eds) (1990) *Successful Aging. Perspectives from the Behavioral Sciences*. New York: Cambridge University Press.

Banks, I. (2002) *MAN: The Haynes Owners Workshop Manual: A Step-by-Step Guide to Men's Health*. Yeovil: Haynes.

Barnes, M. (1997) *Care, Communities and Citizens*. Harlow: Longman.

Barnes, M. and Bennet, G. (1997) *'If They Would Listen ...' An Evaluation of the Fife User Panels*. Edinburgh: Age Concern Scotland.

Barnes, M. and Walker, A. (1996) Consumerism versus empowerment: a principled approach to the involvement of older service users, *Policy and Politics*, 24(4): 375–93.

Barot, R. (ed.) (1996) *The Racism Problematic: Contemporary Sociological Debates on Race and Ethnicity*. Lewiston: Edwin Mellen Press.

Bauman, Z. (1998) *Work, Consumerism and the New Poor*. Buckingham: Open University Press.

Bengtson, V.L. and Robertson, J.F. (eds) (1985) *Grandparenthood*. Beverley Hills: Sage.

Bennett, N., Jarvis, L., Rowlands, O., Singleton, N. and Hasleden, L.

(1996) *Living in Britain: Results from the 1994 General Household Survey.* London: HMSO.

Berghman, J. (1997) The resurgence of poverty and the struggle against exclusion: a new challenge for social security?, *International Social Security Review*, 501: 3–23.

Bernard, M., Phillips, J., Machin, L. and Harding Davies, V. (2000) *Women Ageing: Changing Identities, Challenging Myths.* London: Routledge.

Berry, J.W. (1992) Acculturation and adaptation in a new society, *International Migration*, 30(1): 69–85.

Berry, J.W. (1997) Immigration, acculturation, and adaptation, *Applied Psychology*, 46(1): 5–34.

Berry, J.W. (2001) A psychology of immigration, *Journal of Social Issues*, 57(3): 615–31.

Betancourt, J.R., Green, A.R., Carrillo, J.E. and Ananeh-Firempong, O. (2003) Defining cultural competence: a practical framework for addressing racial/ethnic disparities in health care, *Public Health Reports*, 118(4): 293–302.

Bhalla, A. and Lapeyre, F. (1997) Social exclusion: towards an analytical and operational framework, *Development and Change*, 28: 13–43.

Bhavnani, R. (1994) *Black Women in the Labour Market: A Research Review.* London: Equal Opportunities Commission.

Birren, J. and Dieckmann, L. (1991) Concepts and content of quality of life in later years: an overview, in J. Birren, J. Lubben, J. Rowe and D. Deutchmann (eds) *The Concept and Measurement of Quality of Life in the Frail Elderly.* London: Academic Press.

Birren, J., Lubben, J., Rowe, J. and Deutchmann, D. (eds) (1991) *The Concept and Measurement of Quality of Life in the Frail Elderly.* London: Academic Press.

Blakemore, K. (1999) International migration in later life: social care and policy implications, *Ageing and Society* 19(6): 761–74.

Blakemore, K. and Boneham, M. (1994) *Age, Race and Ethnicity: A Comparative Approach.* Milton Keynes: Open University Press.

Blane, D., Wiggins, R., Higgs, P. and Hyde, M. (2002) *Inequalities in Quality of Life in Early Old Age.* GO Findings No.9. Sheffield: Growing Older Programme.

Blumer, H. (1969) *Symbolic Interactionism: Perspectives and Methods.* Englewood Cliffs, NJ: Prentice Hall.

Bond, J. and Carstairs, V. (1982) *The Elderly in Clackmannan.* Scottish Health Services Studies no. 42. Edinburgh: Scottish Home and Health Department.

Bornat, J., Dimmock, B. and Peace, S.M. (1998) *The Impact of Family Change on Older People: The Case of Step-families.* Research Results, ESRC Population and Household Change Programme.

Bourdieu, P. (1977) *Outline of a Theory of Practice.* Cambridge: Cambridge University Press.

Bowlby, J. (1953) *Child Care and the Growth of Love.* Harmondsworth: Penguin.

Bowling, A. (1991) *Measuring Health: A Review of Quality of Life Measurement Scales.* Buckingham: Open University Press.

Bowling, A. (1995a) 'What things are important in people's lives? A survey of the public's judgements to inform scales of health related quality of life', *Social Science and Medicine,* 41 (10): 1447–62.

Bowling, A. (1995b) 'The most important things in life. Comparisons between older and younger population age groups by gender. Results from a national survey of the public's judgements', *International Journal of Health and Science,* 6: 169–75.

Bowling, A. (1996) The effects of illness on quality of life, *Journal of Epidemiology and Community Health,* 50: 149–55.

Bowling, A. (1997) *Measuring Health: A Review of Quality of Life Measurement Scales,* 2nd edn. Philadelphia: Open University Press.

Bowling, A. (1998) Measuring health-related quality of life among older people, *Aging and Mental Health,* 2(1): 5–6.

Bowling, A. (2001) *Measuring Disease. A Review of Disease Specific Quality of Life Measurement Scales.* 2nd edn. Buckingham: Open University Press.

Bowling, A. and Gabriel, Z. (2004) 'An integrated model of quality of life', *Social Indicators Research.* (In press, to be published autumn 2004).

Bowling, A., Farquhar, M. and Browne, P. (1991) Life satisfaction and associations with social networks and support variables in three samples of elderly people, *International Journal of Geriatric Psychiatry,* 6: 549–66.

Bowling, A., Bannister, D., Sutton, S., Evans, O. and Windsor, J. (2002) A multidimensional model of the quality of life in older age, *Ageing and Mental Health,* 6(4): 355–71.

Bowling, A., Gabriel, Z., Dykes, J., Marriott-Dowding, L., Fleissig, A., Evans, O., Banister, D. and Sutton, S. (2004) Let's ask them: definitions of quality of life and its enhancement among people aged 65 and over, *International Journal of Aging and Human Development*, 56: 269–306.

Boyatzis, R. (1998) *Transforming Qualitative Information*. Thousand Oaks, CA: Sage.

Bradburn, N.M. (1969) *The Structure of Psychological Well-Being*. Chicago: Aldine.

Bradshaw, J., Williams, J., Levitas, R. et al. (2000) The relationship between poverty and social exclusion in Britain. Paper presented to the 26th General Conference of International Association for Research in Income and Wealth, Cracow, 27 August–2 September.

Brau, A. (1996) *Cartographies of Diaspora: Contrasting Identities*. London: Routledge.

Bridgwood, A., Lilly, R., Thomas, M. et al. (2000) *Living in Britain: Results from the 1998 General Household Survey*. London: The Stationery Office.

Brod, M., Stewart, A., Sands, L. and Walton P. (1999) Conceptualization and measurement of quality of life in dementia: the dementia quality of life instrument (DQuality of life), *The Gerontologist*, 39(1): 25–35.

Brodie, J. (1996) *Perspectives on Poverty and Ethnic Minority Elders*. London: Age Concern.

Brown, G. and Harris, T. (1978) *The Social Origins of Depression*. London: Tavistock.

Browne, J.P., O'Boyle, C.A., McGee, H.M., Joyce, R.B., McDonald, N.J., O'Malley, K. and Hiltbrunner, B. (1994) Individual quality of life in the healthy elderly, *Quality of Life Research*, 3: 235–44.

Bruce, E., Surr, C. and Tibbs, M.A. (2002) *A Special Kind of Care: Improving Well-being in People Living with Dementia*. Derby: MHA Care Group.

Bryan, B., Dadzie, S. and Scafe, S. (1985) *The Heart of the Race: Black Women's Lives in Britain*. London: Virago.

Burchardt, T. (2000) Social exclusion: concepts and evidence, in D. Gordon and P. Townsend (eds) *Breadline Europe: The Measurement of Poverty*, Bristol: Policy Press, pp. 385–405.

Burchardt, T., Le Grand, J. and Piachaud, D. (1999) Social exclusion in Britain 1991–1995, *Social Policy and Administration*, 33(3): 227–44.

Burchardt, T., Le Grand, J. and Piachaud, D. (2002a) Introduction, in J. Hills, J. Le Grand and D. Piachaud (eds) *Understanding Social Exclusion*. Oxford: Oxford University Press, pp. 1–12.

Burchardt, T., Le Grand, J. and Piachaud, D. (2002b) Degrees of exclusion: developing a dynamic, multidimensional measure, in J. Hills, J. Le Grand and D. Piachaud (eds) *Understanding Social Exclusion*. Oxford: Oxford University Press.

Burgess, S. and Propper, C. (2002) The dynamics of poverty in Britain, in J. Hills, J. Le Grand and D. Piachaud (eds) *Understanding Social Exclusion*. Oxford: Oxford University Press, pp. 44–61.

Burholt, V. and Wenger, G.C. (1998) Differences over time in older people's relationships with children and siblings, *Ageing and Society*, 18(5): 537–62.

Burholt, V. and Wenger, G.C. (2001) Differences over time in older people's relationships with children, grandchildren, nieces and nephews in rural North Wales, *Ageing and Society*, 21(5): 567–90.

Bury, M. and Holme, A. (1990) Researching very old people, in S. Peace (ed.) *Researching Social Gerontology*. London: Sage, pp. 129–42.

Butt, J. and Mirza, K. (1996) *Social Care and Black Communities*. London: HMSO.

Byrne, D. (1999) *Social Exclusion*. Buckingham: Open University Press.

Bytheway, B. (1995) *Ageism*. Buckingham: Open University Press.

Bytheway, B. (1997) Talking about age: the theoretical basis of social gerontology, in A. Jamieson, S. Harper and C. Victor (eds) *Critical Approaches to Ageing and Late Life*. Buckingham: Open University Press.

Calman K.C. (1983) Quality of life in cancer patients – a hypothesis, *Journal of Medical Ethics*, 10: 124–7.

Cannon, L.W., Higginbotham, E. and Leung, M.L.A. (1991) Race and class bias in qualitative research on women, in J. Lober and S.A. Farrell (eds) *The Social Construction of Gender*. London: Sage.

Carp, F.M. (1987) Environment and aging, in D. Stokols and I. Altman (eds) *Handbook of Environmental Psychology*. New York: Wiley.

Carp, F.M. (1994) Assessing the environment, in M.P. Lawton and J.A. Teresi (eds) *Focus on Assessment Techniques, Annual Review of Gerontology and Geriatrics*, 14: 302–23.

Carp, F.M. and Carp, A. (1984) A complementarity/congruence model of well-being or mental health for the community elderly, in I. Altman, M.P. Lawton and J. Wohlwill (eds) *Elderly People and the Environment*. New York: Plenum, pp. 279–336.

Carr, A.J., Gibson, B. and Robinson, P.G. (2001) Measuring quality of life: is quality of life determined by expectations or experience?, *British Medical Journal*, 322(7296): 1240–43.

Chappell, N.L. (1992) *Social Support and Ageing*. Toronto: Butterworths.

Chappell, N. and Blandford, A. (1991) Informal and formal care: exploring the complementarity, *Ageing and Society*, 11(3): 299–317.

Cherlin, A.J. and Furstenberg, F.F. (1986) *The New American Grandparent: A Place in the Family, A Place Apart*. New York: Basic Books.

Clarke, L. (1992) 'Children's family circumstances: recent trends in Great Britain', *European Journal of Population*, 20(4): 309–40.

Clarke, L., Joshi, H., Di Salvo, P. and Wright, J. (1997) *Stability and Instability in Children's Lives: Longitudinal Evidence from Two British Sources*, Centre for Population Studies Research Paper no. 97–1. London: Centre for Population Studies.

Clarke, L., Joshi, H. and Di Salvo, P. (2000) Children's family change: reports and records of mothers, fathers and children compared, *Population Trends*, 102: 24–33.

Clarke, L. and Cairns, H. (2001) 'Grandparents and the care of children: the research evidence', in B. Broad (ed.) *Kinship Care: The Placement Choice for Children and Young People*. London: Russell House Publishing.

Clarke, L. and Roberts, C. (2002) 'Policy and rhetoric: the growing interest in fathers and grandparents in Britain', in A. Carling, S. Duncan, and R. Edwards (eds) *Analysing Families: Morality and Rationality in Policy and Practice*. London: Routledge, pp. 165–82.

Cohen, S. and Wills, T.A. (1985) Stress, social support, and the buffering hypothesis, *Psychological Bulletin*, 98(2): 310–57.

Cole, D. and Utting, W. (1962) *The Economic Circumstances of Old People*. Welwyn: Codicote Press.

Collopy, B.J. (1988) Autonomy in long-term care: some crucial distinctions, *The Gerontologist*, 28 (supplement): 10–17.

Cooper, H., Arber, S., Daly, T., Smaje, C. and Ginn, M. (2000) *Ethnicity, Health and Health Behaviour: A Study of Older Age Groups*. London: Health Development Agency.

Cooper, M. and Sidell, M. (1994) *Lewisham Older Women's Health Survey*. London: EdROP The City Lit.

Cordingley, L., Hughes, J. and Challis, D. (2001) *Unmet Need and Older People: Towards a Synthesis of User and Provider Views*. York: Joseph Rowntree Foundation.

Courtney, W.H. (2000) Constructions of masculinity and their influence on men's well-being: a theory of gender and health, *Social Science and Medicine*, 50: 1385–401.

Cunningham-Burley, S. (1985) Constructing grandparenthood: anticipating appropriate action, *Sociology*, 19(3): 421–36.

Cunningham-Burley, S. (1986) Becoming a grandparent, *Ageing and Society*, 6: 453–70.

Cunningham-Burley, S. (1987) The experience of grandfatherhood, in C. Lewis and M. O'Brien (eds) *Reassessing Fatherhood: New Observations on Fathers and the Modern Family*. London: Sage.

Cvitkovich, Y. and Wister, A. (2002) Bringing in the life course: a modification to Lawton's ecological model of aging, *Journal of Aging*, 4(1): 15–29.

Darton, D. and Strelitz, J. (eds) (2003) *Tackling UK Poverty and Disadvantage in the Twenty-first Century*. York: Joseph Rowntree Foundation.

Davidson, K. (1999) *Gender, Age and Widowhood: How Older Widows and Widowers Differently Realign Their Lives*. Guildford: University of Surrey.

Davidson, K. and Arber, S. (2003) Older men's health: a lifecourse issue? *Men's Health Journal*, 2(3): 72–5.

Davidson, K., Arber, S. and Ginn, J. (2000) Gendered meanings of care work within late life marital relationships, *Canadian Journal on Aging*, 19(4): 536–53.

Davies, M., Falkingham, J., Love, H. et al. (1998) *Next Generation*. London: Henley Centre.

Dean, M. (2003) *Growing Older in the 21st Century*. Swindon: ESRC.

de Jong Gierveld, J. (1999) A review of loneliness: concepts and definitions, causes and consequences, *Reviews in Clinical Gerontology*, 8: 73–80.

de Jong Gierveld, J. and Kamphuis, F. (1985) The development of a Rasch-type loneliness scale, *Applied Psychological Measurement*, 9(3): 289–99.

de Jong Gierveld, J. and van Tilburg, T. (1999) *Manual of the Loneliness Scale 1999*. Amsterdam: Department of Social Research Methodology, Free University of Amsterdam (updated version 18.01.02).

Dench, G. and Ogg, J. (2002) *Grandparenting in Britain: A Baseline Study*. London: Insitute of Community Studies.

Dench, G., Ogg, J. and Thomson, K. (1999) The role of grandparents, in R. Jowell, J. Curtice, A. Park and K. Thomson (eds) *British Social Attitudes: The 16th Report*. Aldershot: Ashgate.

Department for Work and Pensions (DWP) (2003) *Households Below Average Income 1994/95–2001/02*. London: The Stationery Office.

Department of the Environment, Transport and the Regions (DETR) (1998) *Updating and Revising the Index of Local Deprivation*. London: The Stationery Office.

Department of the Environment, Transport and the Regions (DETR) (2000) *Index of Deprivation, 2000*, regeneration research summary, no. 31. London: DETR.

Department of Health (DoH) (1998a) *Independent Inquiry into Inequalities in Health Report*. London: The Stationery Office.

Department of Health (DoH) (1998b) *Modernising Social Services. Promoting Independence, Improving Protection, Reviewing Standards*, Cm 4169. London: The Stationery Office.

Department of Health (DoH) (2001) *National Framework for Older People*. London: DoH.

Department of Health (DoH) (2002) *Fair Access to Care Services: Guidance on Eligibility Criteria for Adult Social Care*. London: DoH.

Department of Health (DoH) (2003) *Care Homes for Older People. National Minimum Standards and the Care Homes Regulations 2001*, 3rd edn. London: The Stationery Office.

Department of Health and Social Services Inspectorate (DOH/SSI) (1989) *Homes are for Living In: A Model of Evaluating Quality of Care Provided and Quality of Life Experienced in Residential Care Homes for Elderly People*. London: HMSO.

Dominelli, L. (1998) Multiculturalism, anti-racism and social work, in C. Williams, H. Soydan and M.R.D. Johnson (eds) *Social Work and Minorities*. London: Routledge, pp. 36–57.

Drew, L.A. and Smith, P.K. (1999) The impact of parental separation/ divorce on grandparent–grandchild relationships, *International Journal of Aging and Human Development*, 48(3): 191–216.

Dubos R. (1959) *Mirage of Health*. New York: Harper.

Ebrahim, S. (1996) Ethnic elder, *British Medical Journal*, 313: 610–13.

Elam, G., Fenton, K., Johnson, A., Nazroo, J. and Ritchie, J. (1999) *Exploring Ethnicity and Sexual Health*. London: SCPR.

Ellaway, A., Wood, S. and MacIntyre, S. (1999) Someone to talk to? The role of loneliness as a factor in the frequency of GP consultations, *British Journal of General Practice*, 49: 363–7.

Erens, B., Primatesta, P. and Prior, G. (2001) *Health Survey for England 1999: The Health of Minority Ethnic Groups*. London: The Stationery Office.

Estes, C. (1979) *The Aging Enterprise*. San Francisco: Jossey Bass.

Evandrou, M. (2000) Social inequalities in later life: the socio-economic position of older people from ethnic minority groups in Britain, *Population Trends*, autumn: 11–18.

Faden, R. and German, P. (1994) Quality of life: considerations in geriatrics, *Clinics in Geriatric Medicine*, 10(3): 541–50.

Falaschetti, E., Malbut, K. and Primatesta, P. (2002) *Health Survey for England 2000. The General Health of Older People and their Use of Health Services*. London: The Stationery Office.

Falkingham, J. (1998) Financial security in later life, in M. Bernard and J. Phillips (eds) *The Social Policy of Old Age*. London: Centre for Policy on Ageing.

Farquhar, M. (1995) 'Elderly people's definitions of quality of life', *Social Science and Medicine*, 41: 1439–46.

Featherstone, M. and Hepworth, M. (1993) Images of ageing, in J. Bond, P. Coleman and S. Peace (eds) *Ageing in Society: An Introduction to Social Gerontology*, 2nd edn. London: Sage.

Fees, B., Martin, P. and Poon, L. (1999) A model of loneliness in older adults, *Journal of Gerontology, Psychological Sciences*, 54b(4): 231–9.

Fenton, S. (1996) Counting ethnicity: social groups and official categories, in R. Levitas and W. Guy (eds) *Interpreting Official Statistics*. London: Routledge.

Finch, B.K. and Vega, W.A. (2003) Acculturation stress, social support, and self-rated health among Latinos in California, *Journal of Immigrant Health*, 5(3): 109–17.

Finch, J. (1989) *Family Obligations and Social Change*. Cambridge: Polity Press.

Finch, J. and Mason, J. (1993) *Negotiating Family Responsibilities*. London: Routledge.

Flick, U. (2002) *An Introduction to Qualitative Research*. London: Sage.

Fru, F. and Glendenning, F. (1988) *Black and Ethnic Elders: Retirement Issues*. Guildford: Pre-retirement Association.

Fry, P.S. (2000) Whose quality of life is it anyway? Why not ask seniors to tell us about it?, *International Journal of Aging and Human Development*, 50: 361–83.

Gans, H.J. (1972) *People and Plans. Essays on Urban Problems and Solutions*. Harmondsworth: Penguin.

Gardner, K. (2002) *Age, Narrative and Migration: The Life Course and Life Histories of Bengali Elders in London*. Oxford: Berg.

Gibson, H.B. (2001) *Loneliness in Later Life*. Basingstoke: Macmillan.

Giddens, A. (1984) *The Constitution of Society: Outline of the Theory of Structuration*. Cambridge: Polity Press.

Giddens, A. (1991) *Modernity and Self-Identity. Self and Society in the Late Modern Age*. Cambridge: Polity Press.

Gilhooly, M., Phillips, L., Gilhooly, K. and Hanlon, P. (2003) *Quality of Life and Real Life Cognitive Functioning*, GO findings no. 15. Sheffield: Growing Older Programme, University of Sheffield.

Gill, T.M. and Feinstein, A.R. (1994) A critical appraisal of quality of life measurements, *Journal of the American Medical Association*, 272: 619–26.

Ginn, J. (2003) *Gender, Pensions and the Lifecourse: How Pensions Need to Adapt to Changing Family Forms*. Bristol: Policy Press.

Glaser, B. and Strauss, A. (1967) *The Discovery of Grounded Theory*. Chicago: Aldine.

Glennerster, H., Lupton, R., Noden, P. and Power, A. (1999) *Poverty, Social Exclusion and Neighbourhood: Studying the Area Bases*, CASE paper no. 22. London: Centre for Analysis of Social Exclusion, London School of Economics.

Goffman, E. (1961) *Asylums*. Harmondsworth: Penguin.

Goffman, E. (1968) *Stigma: Notes on the Management of Spoiled Identity*. Harmondsworth: Penguin.

Goodwin, R. and Cramer, D. (2002) Marriage and social support in a British–Asian community, *Journal of Community and Applied Social Psychology*, 10(1): 49–62.

Gordon, D., Adelman, L., Ashworth, K. et al. (2000) *Poverty and Social Exclusion in Britain*. York: Joseph Rowntree Foundation.

Gottlieb, B.H. (1985) Social networks and social support: an overview of research, practice, and policy implications, *Health Education Quarterly*, 12(1): 5–22.

Government Actuary's Department (2001) *Marital Projections: England and Wales 12 November 2002*. London: The Stationery Office.

Grewal, I., Nazroo, J., Bajekal, M., Blane, D. and Lewis, J. (2004) Influences on quality of life: a qualitative investigation of ethnic differences among older people in England. *Journal of Ethnic and Migration Studies*, in press.

Grundy, E., Murphy, M. and Shelton, N. (1999) Looking beyond the household: intergenerational perspectives on living kin and contacts with kin in Great Britain, *Population Trends* 97: 19–27.

Gubrium, J. (1995) Voice, context and narrative in aging, *Canadian Journal on Aging*, 14 (S1): 68–81.

Gurney, C. and Means, R. (1993) The meaning of home in later life, in S. Arber and M. Evandrou (eds) *Ageing, Independence and the Life Course*. London: Jessica Kingsley.

Hammersley, M. and Atkinson, P. (1995) *Ethnography: Principles in Practice*, 2nd edn. London: Routledge.

Hancock, R. and Weir, P. (1994) *More Ways than Means: A Guide to Pensioners' Incomes in Great Britain*. London: Age Concern Institute of Gerontology, King's College London.

Hanmer, J. and Hearn, J. (1999) Gender and welfare research, in F. Williams, J. Popay and A. Oakley (eds) *Welfare Research: A Critical Review*. London: UCL Press.

Hanson, J. (2001) From sheltered housing to lifetime homes: an inclusive approach to housing, in S. Winters (ed.) *Lifetime Housing in Europe*. Leuven: Hoger Institut voor de Arbeid.

Hanson, J., Kellaher, L. and Karmona, S. (forthcoming) *Redefining Domesticity*. London: The Housing Corporation.

Harper, S. (1987) The kinship network of the rural aged: a comparison of the indigenous elderly and the retired immigrant, *Ageing and Society*, 7(3): 303–27.

Hazan, H. (1980) *The Limbo People*. London: Routledge and Kegan Paul.

Hazan, H. (1994) *Old Age: Constructions and Deconstructions*. Cambridge: Cambridge University Press.

Hearn, J. (1998) The welfare of men?, in J. Popay, J. Hearn and J. Edwards (eds) *Men, Gender Divisions and Welfare*. London: Routledge, pp. 12–36.

Helgeson, V.S. (2003) Social support and quality of life, *Quality of Life Research*, 12 (supplement 1): 25–31.

Hennessy, C.H. and Hennessy, M. (1990) Community-based long-term care for the elderly: evaluation practice reconsidered, *Medical Care Review*, 47: 221–59.

Heywood, F., Pate, A., Galvin, J. and Means, R. (1999) *Housing Options for Older People*. London: The Housing Corporation.

Hickey, A., O'Boyle, C.A., McGee, H.M. and Joyce, C.R.B. (1999) The schedule for the evaluation of individual quality of life, in C.R.B. Joyce, C.A. O'Boyle and H. McGee (1999) *Individual Quality of Life. Approaches to Conceptualisation and Assessment*. Den Haag: Haywood.

Higgs, P. (1999) Quality of life and changing parameters of old age, *Ageing and Mental Health*, 3(3:) 197–8.

Higgs, P., Hyde, M., Wiggins, R. and Blane, D. (2003) Researching quality of life in early old age: the importance of the sociological dimension, *Social Policy and Administration*, 37(2): 239–52.

Hillier, W. and Hanson, J. (1977) *The Social Logic of Space*. Cambridge: Cambridge University Press.

Hills, J. (1995) *Income and Wealth Vol. 2: A Summary of the Evidence*. York: Joseph Rowntree Foundation.

Hills, J. (1998) *Income and Wealth: The Latest Evidence*, York: Joseph Rowntree Foundation.

Hills, J., Le Grand, J. and Piachaud, D. (eds) (2002) *Understanding Social Exclusion*. Oxford: Oxford University Press.

Hockey, J. (1999) The ideal of home: domesticating the institutional space of old age and death, in T. Chapman and J. Hockey (eds) *Ideal Homes? Social Change and Domestic Life*. London: Routledge.

Hockey, J. and James, A. (2003) *Social Identities and the Life Course*. London: Palgrave.

Hofstede, G. (1980) *Culture's Consequences: International Differences in Work Related Values*. Beverly Hills, CA: Sage.

Holland, C. (2001) Housing histories: the experience of older women across the life course. Unpublished PhD thesis, Open University.

Holmen, K. and Furukawa, H. (2002) Loneliness, health and social network among elderly people – a follow-up study, *Archives of Gerontology and Geriatrics*, 35(3): 261–71.

Home Office (1998) *Supporting Families. A Consultation Document.* London: The Stationery Office.

Hornquist, J.O. (1982) The concept of quality of life, *Scandinavian Journal of Social Medicine*, 10: 57–61.

House of Commons (2003) *The Future of UK Pensions. Work and Pensions Committee, Third Report of Session 2002–03*, Vol. 1. London: The Stationery Office.

Howarth, C., Kenway, P., Palmer, G. and Miorelli, R. (1999) *Monitoring Poverty and Social Exclusion 1999.* York: Joseph Rowntree Foundation.

Howell, S.C. (1983) The meaning of place in old age, in G.D. Rowles and R.J. Ohta (eds) *Aging and Milieu: Environmental Perspectives in Growing Old.* New York: Academic Press, pp. 97–107.

Hubbard, G., Tester, S. and Downs, M. (2001) Family carers talk about their perceptions of nursing homes, *Journal of Dementia Care*, 9(5): 37.

Hubbard, G., Cook, A., Tester, S. and Downs, M. (2002) Beyond words: older people with dementia using and interpreting non-verbal behaviour, *Journal of Aging Studies*, 16(2): 155–67.

Hubbard, G., Cook, A., Tester, S. and Downs, M. (2003a) *Sexual Expression in Institutional Care Settings: An Interactive Multi-media CDROM.* Stirling: University of Stirling, Department of Applied Social Science.

Hubbard, G., Downs, M. and Tester, S. (2003b) Including older people with dementia in research: challenges and strategies, *Aging and Mental Health*, 7(5): 351–62.

Hubbard, G., Tester, S. and Downs, M. (2003c) Meaningful social interactions between older people in institutional care settings, *Ageing and Society*, 23(1): 99–114.

Hunt, A. (1978) *The Elderly at Home.* London: HMSO.

Hunt, S.M. (1997) The problem of quality of life, *Quality of Life Research*, 6: 205–12.

Hyde, M., Wiggins, R.D., Higgs, P. and Blane, D.B. (2003) A measure of quality of life in early old age: the theory, development and properties of a needs satisfaction model (CASP-19), *Ageing and Mental Health*, 7(3): 186–94.

Jagger, C. and Matthews, F. (2002) Gender differences in life expectancy free of impairment at older ages, in S.B. Laditka (ed.) *Health Expectations for Older Women: International Perspectives*. London: Howarth Press.

Janevic, M.R. and Connell, C.M. (2001) Racial, ethnic, and cultural differences in the dementia caregiving experience: recent findings, *The Gerontologist*, 41(3): 334–47.

johnnycash.com (2003) *Johnny and June. http://www.johnnycash.com/june/johnny2.html* (accessed 20 Sept. 2003).

Johnson, C. (1985) Grandparenting options in divorcing families: an anthropological perspective, in V.L. Bengtson and J.F. Robertson (eds) *Grandparenthood*. London: Sage.

Jones, D., Victor, C.R. and Vetter, N. (1982) The problems of loneliness in the community, *Journal of the Royal College of General Practitioners*, 35: 136–9.

Jones, S. (1985) The analysis of depth interviews, in R. Walker (ed.) *Applied Qualitative Research*. Aldershot: Gower.

Joyce, C.R.B., McGee H.M. and O'Boyle, C.A. (1999) Individual quality of life: review and outlook, in C.R.B Joyce, C.A. O'Boyle and H. McGee *Individual Quality of Life. Approaches to Conceptualisation and Assessment*. Den Haag: Haywood.

Kahana, E. (1982) A congruence model of person–environment interaction, in M.P Lawton, P.G. Windley and T.O. Byerts (eds) *Aging and the Environment: Theoretical Approaches*, New York: Springer, pp. 97–121.

Kahana, B. and Kahana, E. (1983) Stress reactions, in P.M. Lewinsohn and L. Teri (eds) *Clinical Geropsychology: New Directions in Assessment and Treatment*. New York: Pergamon Press, pp. 139–69.

Kalache, A. (2000) Men, ageing and health, *The Aging Male*, 3(1): 3–36.

Kalache, A. (2002) Gender-specific health care in the 21st century: a focus on developing countries, *The Aging Male*, 5(3): 129–38.

Kart, C.S. and Ford, M E. (2002) Exploring the factorial structure of the EORTC QLQ-C30: racial differences in measuring health-related quality of life in a sample of urban, older adults, *Journal of Aging and Health*, 14(3): 399–421.

Katbamna, S. and Bakta, P. with Parker, G., Ahmad, W. and Baker, R. (1998) *Experiences and Needs of Carers from the South Asian Communities*. Leicester: Nuffield Community Care Studies Unit.

Kellaher, L. (1998) When and how do institutions work: the caring in homes initiative, in R. Jack (ed.) *Residential versus Community Care: The Role of Institutions in Welfare Provision*. Basingstoke: Macmillan.

Kellaher, L. (2000) *A Choice Well Made: Mutuality as a Governing Principle in Residential Care*. London: Centre for Policy on Ageing.

Kellaher, L., Peace, S. and Willcocks, D. (1990) Triangulating data, in S. Peace (ed.) *Researching Social Gerontology*. London: Sage.

Kelly, M. (2001) Lifetime homes, in S.M. Peace and C. Holland (eds) *Inclusive Housing in an Ageing Society: Innovative Approaches*. Bristol: Policy Press, pp. 55–76.

Kempson, E. and Whyley, C. (1999) *Kept Out or Opted Out? Understanding and Combating Financial Exclusion*. York: Policy Press in association with the Joseph Rowntree Foundation.

Kessel, F., Rosenfield, P.L. and Anderson, N.B. (2003) *Expanding the Boundaries of Health and Social Science: Case Studies in Interdisciplinary Innovation*. Oxford: Oxford University Press.

Kim, J.O. and Mueller, C.W. (1979) *Factor Analysis, Statistical Methods and Practical Issues*. London: Sage.

Kimmel, M. and Messner, M. (2001) *Men's Lives*, Boston, MA: Allyn and Bacon.

King, R., Warnes, A.M. and Williams, A.M. (2000) *Sunset Lives: British Retirement Migration to the Mediterranean*. Oxford: Berg.

Kinsella, K. (1997) The demography of an aging world, in J. Sokolowsky (ed.) *The Cultural Context of Aging*. Washington, DC: Greenwood Press.

Kitwood, T. (1997) *Dementia Reconsidered*. Buckingham: Open University Press.

Knights, D. and Midgley, R. (1998) *User Involvement in Community Care. Where Next in Sheffield?* Sheffield: Sheffield Joint Consultative Committee.

Koskinen, S. (2002) The village community as a resource for the aged. Paper presented to the BSG Annual Conference 2002, Active Ageing: Myth or Reality?, Birmingham.

Kovach, S. and Robinson, J. (1996) The roommate relationship for the elderly nursing home resident, *Journal of Social and Personal Relationships*, 13(4): 627–34.

Kuh, D. and Ben-Shlomo, Y. (1997) *A Life Course Approach to Chronic Disease Epidemiology*. Oxford: Oxford University Press.

Kyriakides, C. and Virdee, S. (2003) Migrant labour, racism and the British National Health Service, *Ethnicity and Health*, 8(4): 283–305.

La Fromboise, T., Coleman, H.L.K. and Gerton, J. (1993) Psychological impact of biculturalism: evidence and theory, *Psychological Bulletin*, 114(3): 395–412.

Larson, R. (1978) Thirty years of research on the subjective well-being of older Americans, *Journal of Gerontology*, 33: 109–25.

Laslett, P. (1989) *A Fresh Map of Life*. London: Weidenfield and Nicholson.

Laws, G. (1994) Contested meanings, the built environment and aging in place, *Environment and Planning*, 26: 1787–802.

Laws, G. (1995) Embodiment and emplacement: identities, representation and landscape in Sun City retirement communities, *International Journal of Aging and Human Development*, 40(4): 253–80.

Laws, G. (1997) Spatiality and age relations, in A. Jamieson, S. Harper and C. Victor (eds) *Critical Approaches to Ageing and Later Life*. Buckingham: Open University Press.

Lawton, M.P. (1972) Assessing the competence of older people, in D.P. Kent, P. Kastenbaum and S. Sherwood (eds) *Research, Planning and Action for the Elderly*. New York: Behavioural Publications.

Lawton, M.P. (1975) The Philadelphia Geriatric Center Morale Scale: a revision, *Journal of Gerontology*, 30: 85–9.

Lawton, M.P. (1980) *Environment and Aging*. Monterey, CA: Brooks/ Cole Publishing.

Lawton, M.P. (1983) Environment and other determinants of well-being in older people, *The Gerontologist*, 23(4): 349–57.

Lawton, M.P. and Nahemow, L. (1973) Ecology and the aging process, in C. Eisdorfer and M.P. Lawton (eds) *The Psychology of Adult Development and Aging*. Washington, DC: American Psychological Association.

Learning Media Unit (LEMU), Sheffield University (2002) *Older Women's Lives and Voices Video*. University of Sheffield: LMU.

Lee, R. (1993) *Doing Research on Sensitive Topics*. London: Sage.

Lefebvre, H. (1991) *The Social Production of Space*. Oxford: Blackwell.

Leisering, L. and Walker, R. (eds) (1998) *The Dynamics of Modern Society*. Bristol: Policy Press.

Lemke, S., Moos, R.H., Mehren, B. and Gauvain, M. (1979) *Multi-*

phasic Environmental Assessment Procedures (MEAP). Handbook for Users. Palo Alto, CA: Social Ecology Laboratory, Veterans Administration, Medical Centre and Stanford University School of Medicine.

Levitas, R. (1998) *The Inclusive Society? Social Exclusion and New Labour.* Basingstoke: Macmillan.

Lieberman, M. (1991) Relocation of the frail elderly, in J. Birren, J. Lubben, J. Rowe and D. Deutchmann (eds) *The Concept and Measurement of Quality of Life in the Frail Elderly.* London: Academic Press.

Lindow, V. (1996) *User Involvement: Community Service Users as Consultants and Trainers.* London: Department of Health.

Litwak, E. (1985) *Helping the Elderly: the Complementary Roles of Informal Networks and Formal Systems.* New York: Guilford Press.

Litwin, H. (1995) The social networks of elderly immigrants: an analytic typology, *Journal of Aging Studies*, 9(2): 155–74.

Lowdell, C., Evandrou, M., Bardsley, M., Morgan, D. and Soljak, M. (2000) *Health of Ethnic Minority Elders in London: Respecting Diversity.* London: Health of Londoners Project.

Lubben, J.E. (1988) Assessing social networks among elderly populations, *Family and Community Health*, 11(3): 42–52.

Lupton, R. and Power, A. (2002) Social exclusion and neighbourhood, in J. Hills, J. Le Grand and D. Piachaud (eds) *Understanding Social Exclusion.* Oxford: Oxford University Press.

McGlone, F., Park, A. and Smith, K. (1998) *Families and Kinship.* London: FPSC.

Mack, M. and Lansley, S. (1985) *Poor Britain.* London: George Allen and Unwin.

McKee, K., Wilson, F., Elford, H., Goudie, F., Chung, M., Bolton, E. and Hinchcliff, S. (2002) *Evaluating the Impact of Reminiscence on the Quality of Life of Older People*, GO Findings no. 8. Sheffield: Growing Older Programme, University of Sheffield.

Madanipour, A., Cars, G. and Allen, J. (eds) (1998) *Social Exclusion in European Cities: Processes, Experiences, and Responses.* London: Jessica Kingsley.

Marcus, C.C. (1995) *House as a Mirror of Self: Exploring the Deeper Meaning of Home.* Berkley, CA: Conari Press.

Marcuse, P. (1996) Space and race in the post-fordist city, in E.

Mingione (ed.) *Urban Poverty and the Underclass: A Reader*. Oxford: Blackwell.

Markides, K.S. and Black, S.A. (1995) Race, ethnicity, and aging: the impact of inequality, in R.H. Binstock and L.K. George (eds) *Handbook of Aging and the Social Sciences*. San Diego: Academic Press, pp. 153–70.

Marshall, V.W. (1995) The state of theory in aging and the social sciences, in R.H. Binstock and L.K. George (eds) *Handbook of Aging and the Social Sciences*. San Diego: Academic Press, pp. 12–30.

Martin, J. and Roberts, C. (1984) *Women and Employment: A Lifetime Perspective*. London: HMSO.

Maslow, A. (1954) *Motivation and Personality*. New York: Harper.

Mason, D. (ed.) (2003) *Explaining Ethnic Differences: Changing Patterns of Disadvantage in Britain*. Bristol: Policy Press.

Mason, J. (1996) *Qualitative Researching*. London: Sage.

Massey, D. (1994) *Space, Place and Gender*. Cambridge: Polity Press.

Mays, N. (1983) Elderly south Asians in Britain: a survey of the relevant literature and themes for future research, *Ageing and Society*, 3: 71–97.

Mills, M. (1997) Narrative identity and dementia: a study of emotion and narrative in older people with dementia, *Ageing and Society*, 17: 673–98.

Mills, M. and Coleman, P. (1994) Nostalgic memories in dementia – a case study, *International Journal of Aging and Human Development*, 38(3): 203–19.

Minkler, M. and Estes, C. (eds) (1999) *Critical Gerontology*. New York: Baywood Press.

Modood, T., Berthoud, R. and Lakey, J. (1997) *Ethnic Minorities in Britain. Diversity and Disadvantage*. London: Policy Studies Institute.

Moos, R.H. and Lemke, S. (1980) Assessing the physical and architectural features of sheltered care settings, *Journal of Gerontology*, 35(2): 75–94.

Moyer, A., Coristine, M., Jamault, M., Roberge, G. and O'Hagan, M. (1999) Identifying older people in need using action research, *Journal of Clinical Nursing*, 8(1): 103–11.

Moynihan, C. (1998) Theories of masculinity, *British Medical Journal*, 317: 1072–5.

Murphy, J. (2003) *Talking Mats ™ and Frail Older People: A Low-tech*

Communication Resource to Help People to Express their Views and Feelings. Stirling: Department of Psychology, University of Stirling.

Nahemow, L. (2000) The ecological theory of aging: Powell Lawton's legacy, in R.L. Rubinstein, M. Moss and M.H. Kleban (eds) *The Many Dimensions of Aging.* New York: Springer, pp. 22–40.

National Action Plan (2001) *United Kingdom National Action Plan on Social Inclusion 2001–2003.* Brussels: European Commission.

Nazroo, J. (2001) *Ethnicity, Class and Health.* London: Policy Studies Institute.

Nazroo, J. (2004) Ethnic disparities in aging health: what can we learn from the United Kingdom? In Critical Perspectives on Racial and Ethnic Differentials in Health in Late Life. N. Anderson, R. Bulatao and B. Cohen (eds.), Washington, D.C.: National Academy Press, in press.

Nazroo, J. (2003) The structuring of ethnic inequalities in health: economic position, racial discrimination and racism, *American Journal of Public Health,* 93(2): 277–84.

Nazroo, J. and Grewal, I. (2002) Qualitative methods for investigating ethnic inequalities: lessons from a study of quality of life among older people, *ESRC Growing Older Programme Newsletter,* 4: 2–3.

Nazroo, J., Bajekal, M., Blane, D., Grewal, I. and Lewis, J. (2003) *Ethnic Inequalities in Quality of Life at Older Ages: Subjective and Objective Components. Research Findings from the Growing Older Programme 11.* www.shef.ac.uk/uni/projects/gop/Nazroo_Findings_11.pdf

Neugarten, B.L., Havighurst, R.J. and Tobin, S.S. (1961) The measurement of life satisfaction, *Journal of Gerontology,* 16: 134–43.

Newsom, J.T., Bookwala, J. and Schulz, R. (1997) Social support measurement in group residences for older adults, *Journal of Mental Health and Ageing,* 3(1): 47–66.

Norbeck, J.S., Lindsey, A.M. and Carrieri, V.L. (1981) The development of an instrument to measure social support, *Nursing Research,* 30(5): September–October: 264–69.

Norman, A. (1985) *Triple Jeopardy: Growing Old in a Second Homeland.* London: Centre for Policy on Ageing.

Noro, A. and Aro, S. (1996) Health-related quality of life among the least dependent institutional elderly compared with the non-institutional elderly population, *Quality of Life Research,* 5: 355–66.

Oakley, A. (1975) *Housewife.* Harmondsworth: Penguin.

O'Boyle, CA. (1997) Measuring the quality of later life. *Philosophy Transactions of the Royal Society of London*, 352: 1871–9.

O'Connor, P. (1994) Salient themes in the life review of a sample of frail elderly respondents in London, *Gerontologist*, 34: 224–30.

Office for National Statistics (ONS) (2002a) *Population: Age, Sex and Legal Marital Status*. London: The Stationery Office.

Office for National Statistics (ONS) (2002b) *Social Focus in Brief: Ethnicity*. London: The Stationery Office.

Oldman, C. and Quilgars, D. (1999) The last resort? Revisiting ideas about older people's living arrangements, *Ageing and Society*, 19(3): 363–84.

OPCS (1996) *General Household Survey: 1993–1994 [computer file]*. Colchester: The Data Archive.

OPCS (1997) *General Household Survey: 1994–1995 [computer file]*. Colchester: The Data Archive.

OPCS (1998) *General Household Survey: 1995–1996 [computer file]*. Colchester: The Data Archive.

OPCS (2000) *General Household Survey: 1998–1999 [computer file]*. Colchester: The Data Archive.

Opportunity for All (2002) *Opportunity for All. Tackling Poverty and Social Exclusion*. London: The Stationery Office.

Oswald, F. (1996) *Hier bin ich zu Hause: Zur Bedeutung des Wohnens: Eine empirische Studie mit gesunden und gehbeeinträchtigten Älteren.* [On the meaning of home: an empirical study with healthy and mobility impaired elders]. Regensburger: Roderer.

Owen, D. (2003) The demographic characteristics of people from minority ethnic groups in Britain, in D. Mason (ed.) (2003) *Explaining Ethnic Differences: Changing Patterns of Disadvantage in Britain*. Bristol: Policy Press.

Parker, G. and Lawton, D. (1994) *Different Types of Care, Different Types of Carer: Evidence from the General Household Survey*. London: HMSO.

Parmelee, P.A. and Lawton, M.P. (1990) Design of special environments for the elderly, in J.E. Birren and K.W. Schaie (eds) *Handbook of Psychology and Aging*, 3rd edn. New York: Academic Press.

Patsios, D. (2001) *Poverty and Social Exclusion Amongst the Elderly*, working paper no. 20, Bristol: Townsend Centre for International Poverty Research, Bristol University.

Peace, S.M. (1977) The elderly in an urban environment: a study of spatial mobility in Swansea. PhD thesis, Department of Geography, University College Swansea.

Peace, S.M. (2002) The role of older people in social research, in A. Jamieson and C. Victor (eds) *Researching Ageing and Later Life*. Buckingham: Open University Press, pp. 226–44.

Peace, S.M. and Holland, C. (eds) (2001) *Inclusive Housing in an Ageing Society: Innovative Approaches*. Bristol: Policy Press.

Peace, S.M., Kellaher, L. and Holland, C. (2003) 'Environment and Identity in Later Life: A Cross Setting Study', End of Award Report L480254011. Swindon: ESRC.

Peace, S.M., Kellaher, L. and Willcocks, D. (1992) *A Balanced Life: A Consumer Study of Residential Life in One Hundred Local Authority Old People's Homes*, research report no. 14. London: Survey Research Unit, Polytechnic of North London.

Peace, S.M., Kellaher, L. and Willcocks, D. (1997) *Re-evaluating Residential Care*. Buckingham: Open University Press.

Phillips, J., Bernard, M., Phillipson, C. and Ogg, J. (2000) Social support in later life: a study of three areas, *British Journal of Social Work*, 30(6): 837–53.

Phillipson, C. (1982) *Capitalism and the Construction of Old Age*. London: Macmillan.

Phillipson, C. (1998) *Reconstructing Old Age*. London: Sage.

Phillipson, C., Bernard, M., Phillips, J. and Ogg, J. (1998) The family and community life of older people: household composition and social networks in three urban areas, *Ageing and Society*, 18(3): 259–89.

Phillipson, C., Bernard, M., Phillips, J. and Ogg, J. (1999) Older people's experiences of community life: patterns of neighbouring in three urban areas, *Sociological Review*, 47(4): 715–43.

Pile, N. and Thrift, N. (eds) (1995) *Mapping the Subject: Geographies of Cultural Transformation*. London: Routledge.

Pinquart, M. and Sörenson, S. (2001) Gender differences in self-concept and psychological well-being in old age: a meta-analysis, *Journals of Gerontology*, 56B: 195–213.

Plummer, K. (1990) Herbert Blumer and the life history tradition, *Symbolic Interaction*, 13(2): 125–34.

Power, A. (2000) *Poor Areas and Social Exclusion*, CASE paper no. 35. London: Centre for Analysis of Social Exclusion, London School of Economics.

Proshansky, H.M., Fabian, A.K. and Kaminoff, R. (1983) Place–identity: physical world socialization of the self, *Journal of Environmental Psychology*, 46: 1097–1108.

Qureshi, H. and Walker, A. (1989) *The Caring Relationship: Elderly People and their Families.* Basingstoke: Macmillan.

Reberger, C., Hall, S. and Criddle, R. (1999) Is hostel care good for you? Quality of life measures in older people moving into residential care, *Australasian Journal of Ageing*, 18(3): 145–9.

Reed, J. and Roskell Payton, V. (1996) Constructing familiarity and managing the self: ways of adapting to life in nursing and residential homes for older people, *Ageing and Society*, 16: 543–60.

Roos, N.P. and Havens, B. (1991) Predictors of successful aging, *American Journal of Public Health*, 81: 63–8.

Rowe, J.W. and Kahn, R.L. (1997) Successful aging, *The Gerontologist*, 37(4): 433–40.

Rowles, G.D. (1978) *Prisoners of Space? Exploring the Geographical Experience of Older People.* Boulder, CO: Westview.

Rowles, G.D. (1983) Geographical dimensions of social support in rural Appalachia, in G.D. Rowles and R.J. Ohta (eds) *Aging and Milieu: Environmental Perspectives on Growing Old.* New York: Academic Press, pp. 111–30.

Rowles, G.D. (1991) Beyond performance: being in place as a component of occupational therapy, *American Journal of Occupational Therapy*, 45: 265–71.

Rowles, G.D. (2000) Habituation and being in place, *Occupational Therapy Journal of Research*, 20(1): 52S–67S.

Rowles, G.D. and Watkins, J.F. (2003) History, habit, heart, and hearth: on making spaces into places, in K.W. Schaie, H.W. Wahl, H. Mollenkopf and F. Oswald (eds) *Aging Independently: Living Arrangements and Mobility.* New York: Springer.

Rubinstein, R.L. (1987) The significance of personal objects to older people, *Journal of Aging Studies*, 4: 131–48.

Rubinstein, R.L. (1989) The home environments of older people: a description of psychosocial processes linking person to place, *Journals of Gerontology*, 44: S45–S53.

Rubinstein, R.L. (1990) Personal identity and environmental meaning in later life, *Journal of Aging Studies*, 4: 131–48.

Rubinstein, R.L. and Parmelee, P.A. (1992) Attachment to place and the representation of the life course by the elderly, in I. Altman and S.M. Low (eds) *Place Attachment*. New York and London: Plenum Press, pp. 139–60.

Rubinstein, R.L., Kilbride, J.C. and Nagy, S. (1992) *Elders Living Alone: Frailty and the Perception of Choice*. New York: Aldine De Gruyter.

Russell, C. and Schofield, T. (1999) Social isolation in old age – a qualitative exploration of service providers' perceptions, *Ageing and Society* 19(1): 69–91.

Russell, D.W. (1996) UCLA Loneliness Scale (version 3) reliability, validity and factor structure, *Journal of Personality Assessment*, 66: 20–40.

Ruth, J.E. and Kenyon, G. (1996) Introduction, *Ageing and Society*, 16(6): 653–8.

Ryan, M.C. and Austin, A.G. (1989) Social supports and social networks in the aged, *IMAGE: Journal of Nursing Scholarship*, 21(3): 176–80.

Scharf, T. and Smith, A.E. (2003) Older people in urban neighbour-hoods: addressing the risk of social exclusion in later life, in C. Phillipson, G. Allan and D. Morgan (eds) *Social Networks and Social Exclusion*. Aldershot: Ashgate.

Scharf, T., Phillipson, C., Kingston, P. and Smith, A.E. (2001) Social exclusion and ageing, *Education and Ageing* 16(3): 303–20.

Scharf, T., Phillipson, C., Smith, A.E. and Kingston, P. (2002a) Older people in deprived areas: perceptions of the neighbourhood, *Quality in Ageing* 3(2): 11–21.

Scharf, T., Phillipson, C., Smith, A.E. and Kingston, P. (2002b) *Growing Older in Socially Deprived Areas: Social Exclusion in Later Life*. London: Help the Aged.

Schuman, J. (1999) The ethnic minority populations of Great Britain – latest estimates, in Office for National Statistics *Population Trends 96*. London: ONS.

Scott, A. and Wenger, G.C. (1995) Gender and social support networks in later life, in S. Arber and J. Ginn (eds) *Connecting Gender and Ageing*. Buckingham: Open University Press, pp. 158–72.

Scottish Executive (2001) *National Care Standards: Care Homes for Older People*. *http://www.scotland.gov.uk/library3/social/chop.pdf* (accessed 2 Dec. 2003).

Seidler, V. (1994) *Unreasonable Men*. New York: Routledge.

Selai, C.E., Elstner, E. and Trimble, M.R. (1999) Quality of life pre and post epilepsy surgery, *Epilepsy Research*, 38(1): 67–74.

Sheldon, J.H. (1948) *The Social Medicine of Old Age*. Oxford: Oxford University Press.

Shelton, N. and Grundy, E. (2000) Proximity of adult children to their parents in Great Britain, *International Journal of Population Geography*, 6(3): 181–95.

Shreeve, M. (2000) Older people in the 21st century. Paper presented to the 'Grandparenting in Britain' conference, London, Family Policy Studies Centre, March.

Sidell, M. (1995) *Health in Old Age: Myth, Mystery and Management*. Buckingham: Open University Press.

Silver, H. (1994) Social exclusion and social solidarity: three paradigms, *International Labour Review*, 133(5–6): 531–78.

Silverman, D. (1993) *Interpreting Qualitative Data: Methods for Analysing Talk, Text and Interaction*. London: Sage.

Silverstein, M. and Long, J.D. (1998) Trajectories of grandparents' perceived solidarity with adult grandchildren: a growth curve analysis over 23 years, *Journal of Marriage and the Family*, 60: 912–23.

Silverstein, M. and Marenco, A.L. (2000) 'Styles of grandparenting: how the Americans enact the grandparenting role', *Journal of Marriage and the Family*.

Sixsmith, A. (1990) The meaning and experience of home in later life, in B. Bytheway and J. Johnson (eds) *Welfare and the Ageing Experience*. Aldershot: Avebury Gower Publishing.

Sixsmith, J. (1986) The meaning of home: an exploratory study of environmental experience, *Journal of Environmental Experience*, 6: 281–98.

Smaje, C. (1995) *Health, 'Race' and Ethnicity: Making Sense of the Evidence*. London: King's Fund Centre/Share.

Smith, A.E., Scharf, T., Phillipson, C. and Sim, J. (2003) *Determinants of quality of life amongst older people in deprived neighbourhoods*, working Paper. Keele: Centre for Social Gerontology, Keele University.

Smith, G. (2003) *Faith in the Voluntary Sector: A Common or Distinctive Experience of Religious Organisations*, working papers in applied social research no. 25. Manchester: University of Manchester.

Social Exclusion Unit (1998) *Bringing Britain Together: A National Strategy for Neighbourhood Renewal*. London: The Stationery Office.

Social Exclusion Unit (2001) *A New Commitment to Neighbourhood Renewal.* London: The Stationery Office.

Social Services Inspectorate (1998) *They Look After Their Own, Don't They? Inspection of Community Care Services for Black and Ethnic Minority Older People.* London: Department of Health.

Soja, E. (1989) *Postmodern Geographies.* London: Verso Press.

Speak, S. and Graham, S. (2000) *Private Sector Service Withdrawal in Disadvantaged Neighbourhoods,* findings no. 230. York: Joseph Rowntree Foundation.

Squires, A. (ed.) (1991) *Multicultural Healthcare and Rehabilitation of Older People.* London: Age Concern England.

Starkey, F. (2003) The 'empowerment' debate: consumerist, professional and liberational perspectives in health and social care, *Social Policy and Society,* 2(4): 273–84.

StatBase (2002) *Population: Age, Sex and Legal Marital Status, 1971 onwards England and Wales: Population Trends 109. www.statistics.gov.uk/STATBASE/xsdataset.asp?v1nk=5753* (accessed 8 Oct. 2002).

Statutory Instrument 2001 no. 3457 (2001) *The Race Relations Act 1976 (Statutory Duties) Order 2001.* London: The Stationery Office. www.hmso.gov.uk/si/si2001/20013458.htm

Stevenson, O. and Parsloe, P. (1993) *Community Care and Empowerment.* York: Joseph Rowntree Foundation.

Strelitz, J. and Darton, D. (2003) Tackling disadvantage: place, in D. Darton and J. Strelitz, (eds) *Tackling UK Poverty and Disadvantage in the Twenty-First Century.* York: Joseph Rowntree Foundation.

Thane, P. (2000) *Old Age in English History: Past Experiences, Present Issues.* Oxford: Oxford University Press.

Thompson, E. (1994) Older men as invisible men, in E. Thompson (ed.) *Older Men's Lives.* Thousand Oaks, CA: Sage, pp. 1–21.

Thornton, P. and Tozer, R. (1994) *Involving Older People in Planning and Evaluating Community Care: A Review of Initiatives.* York: SPRU, University of York.

Thornton, P. and Tozer, R. (1995) *Having a Say in Change. Older People and Community Care.* York: Joseph Rowntree Foundation.

Tijhuis, M.A., de Jong-Gierveld, J., Festiens, E.J. and Kromhout, D. (1999) Changes in and factors related to loneliness in men, The Lutphen Elderly Study: *Age and Ageing,* 28(5): 491–5.

Tinker, A. (1997) *Older People in Modern Society*, 4th edn. London: Longman.

Tornstam, L. (1994) Gero-transcendence: a theoretical and empirical exploration, in L.E. Thomas and S.A. Eisenhandler (eds) *Aging and the Religious Dimension*. Westport, CO: Greenwood, pp. 203–25.

Townsend, P. (1957) *The Family Life of Old People: An Inquiry in East London*. London: Routledge and Kegan Paul.

Townsend, P. (1968) Isolation and loneliness, in E. Shanas, P. Townsend, D. Wedderburn et al. (eds) *Old People in Three Industrial Societies*. London: Routledge and Kegan Paul, pp. 258–88.

Townsend, P. (1979) *Poverty in the United Kingdom*. Harmondsworth: Penguin.

Townsend, P. (1981) The structured dependency of the elderly: the creation of policy in the twentieth century, *Ageing and Society* 1(1): 5–28.

Townsend, P. and Wedderburn, D. (1965) *The Aged in the Welfare State*. London: Bell.

Triandis, H.C. (2001) Individualism–collectivism and personality, *Journal of Personality*, 69(6): 907–24.

Triandis, H.C., Leung, K., Villareal, M.J. and Clack, F.L. (1985) Allocentric versus idiocentric tendencies: convergent and discriminant validation, *Journal of Research in Personality*, 19(4): 395–15.

Triandis, H.C., Bontempo, R., Villareal, M.J., Asai, M. and Lucca, N. (1988) Individualism and collectivism: cross-cultural perspectives on self–ingroup relationships, *Journal of Personality and Social Psychology*, 54(2): 323–38.

Troll, L.E. (1985) The contingencies of grandparenting, in L.M. Burton and V.L. Bengtson (eds) *Grandparenthood*. London: Sage.

Tunaley, J. (1998) Grandparents and the family: support versus interference. Paper presented to the BPS conference, 15 December.

Tunstall, J. (1966) *Old and Alone*. London: Routledge and Kegan Paul.

Uhlenberg, P. and Hammil, B.G. (1998) Frequency of grandparent contact with grandchild sets: six factors that make a difference, *The Gerontologist*, 38(3): 276–85.

Victor, C.R., Henderson, L.M. and Lamping, D.L. (1999) Evaluating the use of standardized health measures with older people: the example of social support, *Reviews in Clinical Gerontology*, 9(4): 371–82.

Victor, C., Scambler, S., Bond, J. and Bowling, A. (2000) Being alone in later life: loneliness, social isolation and living alone, *Reviews in Clinical Gerontology*, 10: 407–17.

Victor, C.R., Scambler, S.J., Shah, S., Cook, D.G., Harris, T., Rink, E. and de Wilde, S. (2002) Has loneliness amongst older people increased? An investigation into variations between cohorts, *Ageing and Society*, 22: 1–13.

Walker, A. (1980) The social creation of poverty and dependence in old age, *Journal of Social Policy*, 9: 49–75.

Walker, A. (1981) Towards a political economy of old age, *Ageing and Society* 1(1): 73–94.

Walker, A. (1993) Poverty and inequality in old age, in J. Bond, P. Coleman and S. Peace (eds) *Ageing in Society*, 2nd edn. London: Sage, pp. 280–303.

Walker, A. (1998) Speaking for themselves: the new politics of old age in Europe, *Education and Ageing*, 13(1): 13–36.

Walker, A. and Hennessy, C. (eds) (2003) *Growing Older Programme – Project Summaries*. Swindon: ESRC.

Walker, A. and Maltby, T. (1997) *Ageing Europe*. Buckingham: Open University Press.

Walker, A. and Walker, C. (1998) Normalisation and 'normal ageing': the social construction of dependency among older people with learning difficulties, *Disability and Society*, 13(1): 125–42.

Walker, A., Maher, J., Coulthard, M., Goddard, E. and Thomas, M. (2001) *Living in Britain. Results from the 2000 General Household Survey*. London: The Stationery Office.

Walker, A., O'Brien, M., Traynor, J. et al. (2002) *Living in Britain: Results from the 2001 General Household Survey*. London: The Stationery Office.

Ward, M. (1997) *Older People and Alcohol: A Literature Review*. London: Health Education Authority.

Ware, J.E.J. and Sherbourne, C.D. (1992) The MOS 36-item short form health survey (SF-36). 1. Conceptual framework and item selection, *Medical Care*, 30(6): 473–83.

Warren, L. (2003) 'Older Women in Sheffield: Lives, Voices and a Video', *Consumers in NHS Research Support Unit NEWS*, Winter/Spring, p.5.

Warren, L. and Maltby, T. (1998) *Older Women in the UK: Their Lives and Their Voices*. Paper presented to the International Sociological Association 14th World Congress, Montreal.

Warren, L., Cook, J. and Maltby, T. (2002) Working with older women from communities in Sheffield, *Growing Older Programme Newsletter*, 4: 3.

Weiss, R. (1973) Loneliness: the experience of emotional and social isolation. Cambridge, MA: MIT Press.

Wenger, G.C. (1984) *The Supportive Network: Coping with Old Age*. London: Allen and Unwin.

Wenger, G.C. (1994) *Support Networks of Older People*. Bangor: Centre for Social Policy Research and Development.

Wenger, G.C. (1983) Loneliness: a problem of measurement, in D. Jerrome (ed.) *Ageing in Modern Society*. Beckenham: Croom Helm, pp. 145–67.

Wenger, G.C. (1992) *Help in Old Age – Facing up to Change*, occasional paper, no. 5. Liverpool: Liverpool University Press.

Wenger, G.C. (1995) A comparison of urban with rural support networks: Liverpool and North Wales, *Ageing and Society*, 15(1): 59–82.

Wenger, G.C. and Burholt, V. (2003) Changes in levels of social isolation and loneliness among older people in rural Wales – a 20 year longitudinal study, *Canadian Journal on Ageing* (in press).

Wenger, G.C. and Tucker, I. (2002) Using network variation in practice: identification of support network type, *Health and Social Care in the Community*, 10(1): 28–35.

Wenger, G.C., Davies, R., Shahtahmasebi, S. and Scott, A. (1996) Social isolation and loneliness in old age: review and model refinement, *Ageing and Society*, 16: 333–58.

Whitehouse, P. (1999) Quality of life in Alzheimer's disease: future directions, *Journal of Mental Health and Aging*, 5(1): 107–11.

Willcocks, D., Peace, S.M. and Kellaher, L. (1987) *Private Lives in Public Places*. London: Tavistock.

Williams, S.W. and Dilworth-Anderson, P. (2002) Systems of social support in families who care for dependent African American elders, *The Gerontologist*, 42(2): 224–36.

Willmott, P. (1986) *Social Networks, Informal Care and Public Policy*. London: Policy Studies Institute.

Wilson, G. (1987) Women's work: the role of grandparents in inter-generational transfers, *Sociological Review*, 35(4): 703–20.

Witzelben, H.D. (1968) On loneliness, *Psychiatry*, 21: 31–43.

Wood, V. and Robertson, J. (1976) The significance of grand-parenthood, in J. Gubrium (ed.) *Times, Roles, and Self in Old Age*. New York: Human Sciences Press.

World Health Organization (WHO) (1993) *Measuring Quality of Life: The Development of the World Health Organization Quality of Life Instrument (WHOQOL)*. Geneva: WHO.

World Health Organization (WHO) (2002) *Active Ageing: A Policy Framework*. Geneva: WHO.

Wu, Z. and Hart, R. (2002) Social and health factors associated with support among elderly immigrants in Canada, *Research on Ageing*, 24(4) 391–412.

Young, M. and Willmott, P. (1957) *Family and Kinship in East London*. London: Routledge and Kegan Paul.

Ziller, R.C. (1974) Self–other orientation and quality of life, *Social Indicators Research*, 1: 301–27.

Zingmark, A., Norberg, K. and Sandman, P.O. (1995) The experience of being at home throughout the life course: investigation of persons 2 to 102, *International Journal of Aging and Human Development*, 41(1): 47–62.

Zukin, S. (1992) *Landscapes of Power: from Detroit to Disney World*. Berkeley: University of California Press.

Index

Page numbers in *italics* refer to tables and figures.

activities, social
  importance for quality of life, 27–8
  within care institutions, 219–20,
    222
  see also civic activities
African populations
  social support, 172–87
  see also ethnic minorities
ageism, experience of female elders,
    158–9, *160–61*
agency (consultation and
    involvement)
  experience of female elders, 155–63
  in care institutions, 216–21
alcohol consumption
  health risk among males, 138–9,
    139, 145, *148*
  statistics, *140*
amenities, local
  contribution to quality of life,
    45–6, *46*
  see also civic activities
Asian populations
  social support, 172–87
  see also ethnic minorities
autonomy
  in care institutions, 213–20
  see also empowerment, social

Bangladeshi populations
  social support, 172–87
  socio-economic inequalities,
    40–57, *41, 42, 44, 46, 47, 48*

see also ethnic minorities
Bangor Longitudinal Study of Ageing
    (BLSA), 170
Barnes, M., and Walker, A., 165
behaviour, health
  among males, 130–47, *131, 138,
    139, 146*
  Growing Older survey, 133–47,
    131, 134
  statistics, *137*
Bengtson, V.L., and Robertson, J.F.,
    193
Berghman, J., 83–4
Better Government for Older People
    (BGOP), 152, 188–9
Blane, D., 4
BLSA (Bangor Longitudinal Study of
    Ageing), 170
Bornat, J., 190
Bourdieu, P., 65
Bowlby, J., 68
Bowling, A., 168
Bradshaw, J., 87
Bristol University, 112
British Nationality Act (1948), 36
British Social Attitudes Survey, 190,
    191
Burchardt, T., 86–7

care homes
  Growing Older quality of life
    survey, 210–24, *222*
Care Standards Act (2000), 210

Caribbean populations
quality of life of female Caribbeans,
150–66
social support, 172–87
socio-economic inequalities,
40–57, *41, 42, 44, 46, 47, 48*
see also ethnic minorities
CASE (Centre for Analysis of Social
Exclusion), 84
*CASP (Control, Autonomy, Self-
realisation and Pleasure) 19*
Scale, 4
Census (2001), 35–7, *36,* 129, 174
Centre for Analysis of Social
Exclusion (LSE), 84
Cheetham, Manchester
deprivation survey, 88–104, *88,
94–6, 97, 102, 103, 104*
Cherlin, A.J., and Furstenberg, F.F.,
193
Chinese populations
frail elders in care institutions,
210–24, *222*
quality of life of female Chinese,
150–66
social support, 172–87
socio-economic inequalities,
40–57, *41, 42, 44, 46, 47, 48*
see also ethnic minorities
civic activities
contribution to quality of life,
45–6, *46*
exclusion from, *95, 96*
see also community work
Clubmoor, Liverpool
deprivation survey, 88–104, *88,
94–6, 97, 102, 103, 104*
Cole, D., and Utting, W., 82
community work
social role, 51–3
see also civic activities

control, in care institutions, 213–20
*Control, Autonomy, Self-realisation
and Pleasure (CASP) 19 Scale,* 4
Cunningham-Burley, S., 199
consultation (agency)
experience of female elders, 155–63
in care institutions, 216–21
crime, statistics, *45*

Dean, M., 4
De Jong Gierveld, J.
and van Tilburg, T., 97
loneliness scale, 97, 109, 110
demographics *see* statistics,
population
Dench, G., 191
deprivation (material and social)
Growing Older survey, 88–104, *88,
94–6, 97, 102, 103, 104*
measures of, 46–7, *46,* 91–3, *92*
past research, 82–3
population characteristics, *91, 92*
see also social exclusion
discrimination, experience of female
elders, 158–9, 160–63
domestic environment
and quality of life, 22–3
relevance in old age, 69–72, 73–4
see also neighbourhood
environment
Drew, L.S., and Smith, P.K., 190–91
'Durkheimian conspiracy' (Levitas), 84

'ecological model' of ageing (Lawton
& Nahemow), 66
economic activity *see* employment
Economic and Social Research
Council (ESRC), 2
economic inequalities
of ethnic groups, 40–57, *41, 42, 44,
46, 47, 48*

employment
  among ethnic groups, 40, 42–3, *42*
  inequalities for ethnic elders,
    57–8
  social role, 50–51, 55–6
empowerment, social
  experience of female elders,
    155–63
  in care institutions, 216–21
environment *see* domestic
    environment; neighbourhood
    environment
environment-person interaction,
    60–80
'environmental press' (Lawton &
    Nahemow), 66
EQUAL (Extend Quality of Life)
    initiative, 2
  see also quality of life
ESRC (Economic and Social Research
    Council), 2
Estes, C., 82
ethnic minorities
  demography, 35–8, *36*
  quality of life of female minorities,
    150–66
  social roles, 49–57
  social support, 170–87
  socio-economic inequalities,
    40–57, *41, 42, 44, 46, 47, 48*
*European Forum on Population Ageing
    Research,* 6
Evandrou, M., 91, *92*, 93
exclusion, social *see* social exclusion
Extend Quality of Life (EQUAL)
    initiative, 2
  see also quality of life

Fair Access to Care Initiative (Dept. of
    Health), 187
Falkingham, J., 82

families
  as social networks, 19–22, 47–8, *47*,
    175–6, 178–81
  effect of family breakdown, 195,
    197
  impact of migration, 57
  importance to elders, 159,
    218–19
  role of elders, 53–4, 55, 197–206
  see also grandparenthood;
    relationships, social
Family Resources Survey (FRS),
    173
females, Growing Older quality of life
    survey, 150–66
Fife User panels Project [Older
    Women's Project], 151
finance
  importance for quality of life,
    29–30
  see also income
'Fourth Age' stage of life (Laslett),
    209
Fourth National Survey of Ethnic
    Minorities (1993–4), 39, 43,
    45–8, 171–2
friends
  role among ethnic elders, 175–6,
    181
  social importance, 20
FRS (Family Resources Survey), 173

Gans, H.J., 86
gardens *see* domestic environment
General Household Survey, 16–17,
    91, 93, 133, 137–9, *137, 138, 139,
    146, 148,* 182
Giddens, A., 65–6
GO Programme *see* Growing Older
    Programme
Gordon, D. et al., 87, 93

Granby, Liverpool
  deprivation survey, 88–104, *88,*
    94–6, 97, 102, 103, 104
grandchild-grandparent relationship,
    20, 195–9, *196,* 203–4
  see also families
grandparenthood
  Growing Older survey, 193–208
  New Labour opinions, 188–9
  past research, 189–92
  responsibilities, 54, 201–3
  symbolic significance, 200–201
  see also families
Growing Older Programme
  future research, 225–9
  history, 2–3
  overview, 3–6
  projects, 3–4, *12–13*
Growing Older Quality of Life
    surveys
  environment-person interaction,
    62–78
  ethnic inequalities, 39–57
  female elders, 150–66
  frail elders in care institutions,
    210–24, *222*
  grandparenthood, 193–208
  health behaviour of male elders,
    133–47
  loneliness & social isolation, 111–26
  poverty & social exclusion, 86–106
  quality of life, 16–32, 150–66
  social support & ethnicity, 172–87
Grundy, E. et al., 191

Hancock, R., and Weir, P., 82
health
  importance for quality of life, 28–9
  inequalities among ethnic groups,
    40, *41,* 58
  psychological wellbeing, 24–6

health services, provision among
    ethnic elders, 181–3
health, male
  behaviour, 130–47, *131, 137, 138,*
    139, 146
  Growing Older survey, 133–47,
    134
  statistics, *137*
Health Survey for England (HSE)
    (1999), 39, 40–43, *41*
Helgeson, V.S., 168
Hillier, W., and Hanson, J., 65
Hills, J., 82
hobbies, importance for quality of
    life, 27–8
Holmen, K., and Fukuwara, H., 124
homes (spatiality) *see* domestic
    environment
homes, care
  Growing Older quality of life
    survey, 210–24, *222*
Housing Options for Older People,
    80
HSE (*Health Survey for England*)
    (1999), 39, 40–43, *41*
ID2000 (*Index of Deprivation, 2000*),
    46–7, *46,* 49
identity, individual
  and environment, 60–80
income, household, 43, *44*
  see also finance
independence, importance for quality
    of life,
    30–32
Index of Deprivation (2000), 46–7, *46,*
    49
Index of Local Deprivation (1998),
    88
Index of Multiple Deprivation
    (Evandrou), 91, *92*

Indian populations
    social support, 172–87
    socio-economic inequalities,
        40–57, *41, 42, 44, 46, 47, 48*
    see also ethnic minorities
'insideness' (biographical concept),
    74–5
institutions, care
    Growing Older quality of life
        survey, 210–24, *222*
isolation, social
    measures of, 96–7, *97*
    see also loneliness

Johnson, C., 193

Kalache, A., 133
Kempson, E., and Whyley, C., 86

Laslett, P., 56–7, 209
Laws, G., 67–8
Lawton, M.P., and Nahemow, L.,
    66
Lefebvre, H., 65
Levitas, R., 84
Lewisham Older Women's Health
    Survey, 151
Lieberman, M., 209
life satisfaction in old age, 24–6
    see also quality of life
Liverpool
    deprivation survey, 88–104, *88,*
        94–6, 97, 102, 103, 104
London
    deprivation survey, 88–104, *88,*
        94–6, 97, 102, 103, 104
    University College, 112
London School of Economics, 84
Longsight, Manchester
    deprivation survey, 88–104, *88,*
        94–6, 97, 102, 103, 104

loneliness
    definition, 108–9, *117,* 120–21
    Growing Older survey, 111–26
    measures of, 96–7, *97,* 109–10
    past research, 110–111
    prevalence, 115–19, *117, 118*
Lubben Social Network Scale, 174

McClemens scoring system
    [household size], 43
males
    Growing Older health &
        partnership survey, 133–47, *134*
    health behaviour, 130–47, *131, 137,*
        138, 139, 146
    health statistics, *137*
    marital status, *148*
Manchester
    deprivation survey, 88–104, *88,*
        94–6, 97, 102, 103, 104
Marcuse, P., 84
marriage
    breakdown, 195, 197
    statistics, *148*
Maslow, A., 14
Massey, D., 65
Men's Health Forum, 132
migration (into UK)
    impact on family relations, 57
    impact on social support
        experiences, 176–7
    statistics, 35–8, *36*
Minkler, M., and Estes, C., 82
minorities, ethnic *see* ethnic
    minorities
money
    importance for quality of life, 29–30
    see also income
Moss Side, Manchester
    deprivation survey, 88–104, *88,*
        94–6, 97, 102, 103, 104

Moynihan, C., 132
multiple exclusion, 101–3, *102, 104*

National Collaboration on Ageing
    Research (NCAR), 228–9
*National Service Framework for Older
    People*, 130, 187
neighbourhood environment
    deprivation, *88*
    impact on quality of life, 22–3, 43,
        45–7, *45*
    relevance in old age, 74–8
    social exclusion, 85–6, *95, 96,*
        100–101
    see also domestic environment
neighbourhood-person interaction,
    60–80
networks, social
    among ethnic elders, 169–70,
        175–6
    families as, 19–22, 47–8, *47,* 175–6,
        178–81, 218–19
    see also relationships, social
Newham, London Borough of
    deprivation survey, 88–104, *88,*
        94–6, 97, 102, 103, 104
New Labour
    definition of social exclusion, 83
    opinions on grandparenthood,
        188–9
Newsom, J.T. et al., 168
Norbeck Social Support
    Questionnaire, 173–4
nursing homes
    Growing Older quality of life
        survey, 210–24, *222*

objects, role in reminiscence, 72–8
occupational status
    ethnic groups, 40, 42–3, *42,*
        57–8

Office for National Statistics (ONS)
    Omnibus Survey, 16, 112–13, 115,
        193–5, 199
Older Women's Lives and Voices
    (OWLV) project, 150–66
Omnibus Survey (ONS), 16, 112–13,
    115, 193–5, 199

Pakistani populations
    socio-economic inequalities,
        40–57, *41, 42, 44, 46, 47, 48*
    see also ethnic minorities
Park, London Borough of Newham
    deprivation survey, 88–104, *88,*
        94–6, 97, 102, 103, 104
Parmelee, P.A., 68–9
participation, community
    among ethnic groups, *48*
    experience of female elders,
        156–8
partnerships
    and quality of life, 129–30
    Growing Older survey, *134*
    statistics, 129
pastimes, importance for quality of
    life, 27–8
patios *see* domestic environment
Peace, S., 4
person-environment interaction,
    60–80
Philadelphia Geriatric Center Morale
    Scale, 80
Phillips. J., 172
Phillipson, C., 82, 172, 190
photographs, role in maintaining
    identity, 72–3
Pirrie, Liverpool
    deprivation survey, 88–104, *88,*
        94–6, 97, 102, 103, 104
'place attachment' model (spatiality),
    68–9

Plashet, London Borough of
    Newham
  deprivation survey, 88–104, *88,*
    94–6, 97, 102, 103, 104
population, white
  socio-economic state, 40–48, *42, 44*
  see also ethnic minorities
population statistics *see* statistics,
    population
possessions, personal
  role in maintaining identity, 72–3
poverty
  Growing Older survey, 86–106
  past research, 82–3
  see also deprivation (material and
    social); social exclusion
Power, A., 85
Prisoners of Space? (Rowles), 67
public services
  exclusion from, *95, 96,* 99–100
  experiences of ethnic women,
    161–3
  provider viewpoint, 164–5
  see also social care services

quality of life
  definition & models, 14–15, *18,* 38,
    129–30
  development of conceptual
    framework, 16–32
  predictors of, 18–19
  see also Growing Older Quality of
    Life surveys
Quality of Life Instrument (World
    Health Organization), 15
Quality of Life Survey (Growing
    Older Programme), 16–32

racism
  experience of female elders, 161–2,
    163

Regulation of Care (Scotland) Act
    (2001), 210
reminiscence, 72–8
relationships, social, 19–22
  among ethnic minorities, 169–70,
    175–6
  exclusion from, *95, 96–8, 96, 97*
  within care institutions, 217–19,
    222
  see also grandparent-grandchild
    relationship; networks, social
religion, role for ethnic elders, 51–3,
    56–7
residential homes
  Growing Older quality of life
    survey, 210–24, *222*
roles (social)
  community work, 51–3
  employment, 50–51, 55–6
  importance for quality of life,
    27–8
  of elders within families, 53–4, 55,
    197–206
  of friends, 175–6, 181
  religion, 51–3, 56–7
Rowe, J.W., and Kahn, R.L., 107
Rowles, G., 67, 74–5, 85
  and Watkins, J.F., 67
Rowntree Foundation, 87
Rubinstein, R.L., 68–9
  and Parmelee, P.A., 68

St Stephens, London Borough of
    Newham
  deprivation survey, 88–104, *88,*
    94–6, 97, 102, 103, 104
Scotland
  quality of life within care
    institutions, 211–21
  social support and ethnicity,
    172–87

'sense of self'
  among frail elders, 213–21, *222*
services, pubic *see* public services
Sheffield
  Better Government for Older
    People, 152
  quality of life of older females,
    149–66
Sheldon, J.H., 107
Silverstein, M.
  and Long, J.D., 193
  and Marenco, A.L., 192
smoking, health behaviour among
  males, 138, *138*, 145
social care services, provision among
  ethnic elders, 181–3
social deprivation *see* deprivation
  (material and social)
social exclusion
  definition, 83–6, 87
  Growing Older Survey, 111–26
  measures of., 91–103, *95, 96, 97, 102*
  see also deprivation (material and
    social); poverty
social isolation
  definition, 108
  measures of, 96–7, *97*
  see also relationships, social
social networks *see* networks, social
social relationships *see* relationships,
  social
social support
  among ethnic elders, 169–72
  definition, 168–9, 174
  families as, 19–22
  Growing Older survey, 172–87
Soja, E., 65
Somali populations
  quality of life of female Somalis,
    150–66
  see also ethnic minorities

Southampton Self-Esteem Scale, 80
space (spatiality), importance in old
  age, 66–72, *73–4*
statistics, population
  ethnic composition, 35–8, *36*
  partnership, *91, 92*, 129, *148*
Stevenson, O., and Parsloe, P., 164
Supporting Families (Home Office),
  188
Surveys *see* Growing Older Quality of
  Life Surveys

'Talking Mats™' (research tool), 4,
  212
'Third Age' roles (Laslett), 56–7
Thompson, E., 127
Townsend, P., 66, 107, 196
  and Wedderburn, D., 82
transportation, impact on quality of
  life, 23–4
Troll, L.E., 193
Tunaley, J., 191
typology
  loneliness in old age, 108–9,
    113–14, 121–3
  social support, 168

UCLA Loneliness Scale, 109
Uhlenberg, P., and Hammil, B.G.,
  193, 197
UN Research Agenda on Ageing, 6
University College, London, 112
urban deprivation *see* deprivation
  (material and social)

voluntary organisations
  social support to ethnic elders,
    183–4
voluntary work, social role, 51–3

Walker, A., 82

Weiss, R., 107
welfare services *see* public services;
   social care services
wellbeing in old age, 24–6
   see also quality of life
Wenger, G.C., 66
'Wheel of Life' (research tool), 4,
   64–5, *64*
Witzelben, H.D., 107

Women, Growing Older quality of
   life survey, 150–66
World Health Organization
   quality of life definition, 129–30
   Quality of Life Instrument, 15

Young, M., and Willmott, P., 196